W9-CAS-443

THE WHAT'S HAPPENING TO MY BODY?
BOOK FOR BOYS

BOOKS BY LYNDA MADARAS

*What's Happening to My Body?: A Growing Up Guide for
Mothers and Daughters* (with Area Madaras)

Womancare: A Gynecological Guide to Your Body (with Jane
Patterson, M.D.)

Woman/Doctor: The Education of Jane Patterson, M.D. (with
Jane Patterson, M.D.)

Great Expectations (with Leigh Adams)

The Alphabet Connection (with Pam Palewicz-Rousseau)

Child's Play

THE WHAT'S HAPPENING TO MY BODY?
BOOK FOR BOYS

A Growing Up Guide for Parents and Sons

LYNDA MADARAS
with DANE SAAVEDRA

Drawings by Jackie Aher

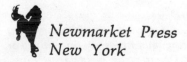

Newmarket Press
New York

Copyright © 1984 Lynda Madaras

This book published simultaneously in the United States of America and in Canada.

All rights reserved. This book may not be reproduced, in whole or in part, in any form, without permission. Inquiries should be addressed to Newmarket Press, 3 East 48th Street, New York, New York 10017

First Edition
1 2 3 4 5 6 7 8 9 0 F/C
      3 4 5 6 7 8 9 0 F/P

Library of Congress Cataloging in Publication Data

Madaras, Lynda.
  The "What's happening to my body?" book for boys.

  Bibliography: p.
  Includes index.
  1. Adolescent boys—Health and hygiene. 2. Puberty.
I. Saavedra, Dane. II. Title.
RJ143.M33 1984   612'.66   84-16667
ISBN 0-937858-39-0
ISBN 0-937858-40-4 (pbk.)

Manufactured in the United States of America

Quantity Purchases

Companies, professional groups, clubs, and other organizations may qualify for special terms when ordering quantities of this title. For information, contact the Special Sales Department, Newmarket Press, 3 East 48th Street, New York, New York 10017. Phone (212) 832-3575.

CONTENTS

LIST OF ILLUSTRATIONS

FOREWORD
by Ralph I. Lopez, M.D.

For the past sixteen years my practice has been devoted solely to the care of teenagers. I begin to see boys and girls when they are twelve and carry them through their college years. Some time ago I had the opportunity to review Lynda Madaras's book *What's Happening To My Body?*, which was geared for girls and which I thought was an ideal book to answer the many questions and concerns of the young girl who is entering puberty. Moreover, it answered these questions in such a way that mothers and daughters—perhaps even fathers and daughters—would be able to converse together about sexual topics. I was delighted, and yet it was evident that a book was needed to answer the same questions for boys. In this new volume, Ms. Madaras fulfills the promise of her first book in making this kind of information available for the young, developing boy.

There is a fascinating assumption on the part of both parents and teenagers today that the kids "know it all" in regard to sex. I take care of boys and girls of all races and religious creeds and of every conceivable economic bracket, who live in a major urban center, and yet I am constantly amazed at the discrepancy between fiction and fact, or myth and reality, where sexual topics are concerned. It is certainly true that our exposure to these topics has increased extraordinarily from my own 1950s teenaged years. So one would expect that the teenagers have much more information available to them. But, alas, we lose sight of the fact that it is the nature of young teens to brag about what they think they know, and to be reluctant to ask what may be the "embarrassing questions." What Ms. Madaras does in her book is answer the "embarrassing questions" with very direct and specific language. She doesn't mince her words and you get a sense that she understands the turmoil of the young teenager who is grasping for answers.

I would strongly urge parents as well as their sons to read Ms. Madaras's book, to get a sense of the questions that teenage boys will ask. As she points out, it is seldom that we get a chance to have that famous "talk" with boys, or girls for that matter. And yet the question that boys are forever asking me is, indeed, "Am I normal?" They ask this about their height, their rate of growth, their hand size and, if they can, about their genitals! What I usually do is give them a sense that indeed all *is* normal. I think that Ms. Madaras's book is must reading, since, as she points out, it will provide the basic information that young boys want and need about what's happening to their bodies.

RALPH I. LOPEZ, M.D.
Associate Professor of Pediatrics and
Attending Physician: Adolescent Clinic,
The New York Hospital–Cornell Medical School

THE WHAT'S HAPPENING TO MY BODY?
BOOK FOR BOYS

INTRODUCTION FOR PARENTS:
Why I Wrote This Book

Toward the end of the school year, I give each of the boys and girls in my sex-education classes a raw egg and a homework assignment that goes something like this.

We're going to play a game. For one week, this egg is your baby. Fortunately for you, you don't have to feed it or change its diapers or get a job in order to earn enough money to buy clothes for it and put a roof over its head. But other than this, you have to take care of the egg as if it really were a baby and you were responsible for it. This means that you can't leave it alone unless you arrange for someone else to watch it while you're gone.

I'm giving you a break, though. I'm going to say that your babies are old enough to sleep through the night. This means that your baby won't wake up at two or three in the morning, howling to be fed—an unfortunate habit that most real babies have during the first months of their lives.

As I say, your babies are old enough to sleep through the night, so all you have to do at bedtime is give baby a kiss

1

and tuck him or her (you decide which it is) into the re-
frigerator. You don't have to worry about baby again until
the next morning. But in the morning, you have to remember to take your baby out of the fridge and bring it to school.

When you forget to bring your lunch money or gym clothes
or math book to school, nothing *too* terrible happens. But if
you forget to bring your baby to school even once, it's dead
and you're out of the game. Not only that, but if any member
of the Child Welfare League finds a neglected baby—that is,
a baby left unattended—that baby will be confiscated.

I am president of the Child Welfare League, and all the staff
and teachers are members. So is every student in the school,
which means that you, too, are a member of the League.
You are sworn to protect the welfare of all egg babies, and as
your president, I expect every member of the League to be
extremely vigilant about confiscating unattended and neglected babies.

At the end of the week, I will take all surviving babies and
their parents out to lunch.

Good luck!

P.S. The parents of confiscated babies will *not* be taken to
lunch.

The egg babies in my classes do not fare well. Most die of
multiple fractures soon after birth. Some rot. Others simply disappear in the eternity of time that is a child's week. Still others
are confiscated by the (at times) alarmingly zealous junior
members of the Child Welfare League.

One year there was even a baby who committed suicide—at
least that's how the baby's "father" attempted to explain the
demise of his egg. It seems this baby had, "all by itself," totally of
its own accord, rolled off his desk in the middle of French class.
The father tried to argue that the parent of a suicidal baby
deserved to be taken out to lunch. Being a hard-hearted lot, the
class refused to acknowledge his point.

So far, in six years of teaching these classes, I have only had to
take two kids and their egg babies out to lunch (and there was

some talk in one case about a fresh egg having been substituted for a broken baby).

I must admit that I get a real kick out of watching what goes on at school in the week during this homework assignment. There are always a couple of boys who try to get one of the girls to care for their babies because "taking care of babies is woman's work." It warms the cockles of my heart to see this tactic fall flat on its face. But there are also the boys who take their parenting very seriously. I'll see them out on the patio at lunch, four or five boys eating together, with their egg babies resting on a strip of soft velvet in the center of the table. They'll be chatting away about the various bumps and cracks their babies have just narrowly escaped, sounding for all the world like the congregations of young mothers who gather over baby strollers in the park to compare notes and trade tales of barely averted childhood disasters.

Within a day or so after I have given the assignment, the egg babies have taken on definite personalities. Carefully crayoned features appear on their formerly blank faces, and the "parents" have all named their babies. Ingenious cribs and cradles and carriages have been fashioned. Once, a boy brought his egg to school in one of those plastic, oval-shaped containers that some panty hose comes in—a "self-contained life-support capsule," the proud father explained. It always surprises me that it is not just the younger kids but also the older teens—and the boys as well as the girls—who get involved in the game and set about designing these cribs and cradles and such for their babies. The sight of a hulking fifteen-year-old with the build of a football player trotting across the campus with his egg baby tenderly tucked in a carefully constructed milk carton cradle never fails to amaze me.

There's always an enterprising young soul, usually a girl, who sets up a baby-sitting service and offers excellent child care for fees ranging from a nickle to twenty-five cents a day. However, she doesn't always offer after-school or night care, and, alas, all too often her charges are dead by the following morning. And, oh, the steely-eyed League members, reprovingly tight-lipped and full of righteous indignation, confiscating the poor egg babies left all alone to fend for themselves in the far reaches of the playing field, or forgotten and abandoned in darkened classrooms at the end of the day. Such devotion to the cause!

This homework assignment comes at the end of a section of the curriculum in which the kids, at least the ones in my older classes, tackle such thorny issues as:

- How old should you be before you have sex?
- How do you know if you're ready for sex?
- Should you wait until you're married?
- How to say no to sex
- Birth control
- The fact that birth control isn't 100 percent effective
- Abortion
- Parenthood
- Sexuality and the responsibility for the lives and feelings of others

The thinking behind the egg baby assignment is, of course, to give kids some idea of the realities of and the responsibilities involved in parenthood. I suppose that at the heart of it, this assignment is really nothing more than an old-fashioned moral object lesson, something along the lines of the stories my grandmother would tell in which children, though warned not to, would skate on thin-ice ponds and drown. Although I heard these tales often, I did venture out on a few thin-ice ponds in my time, and, all in all, the warnings did not have a profound effect on me. So I am not naive enough to think that giving kids raw eggs to take care of for a week is going to make them stop in the middle of the throes of teenage passion and think about forgoing sex altogether or at least using birth control. Still, I figure it can't hurt. We do, after all, have a virtual epidemic of teenage pregnancies in this country, over a million babies born to teenage mothers each year. One-half of today's teenagers, some 11 million kids, are sexually active. Four out of every ten of today's fourteen-year-old girls will become pregnant at least once during their teenage years. Given these facts, anything—even a long shot like the egg baby assignment—seems worth a try.

Even if this assignment never prevents a single teenage pregnancy, the kids have fun and I like to think they learn something from it. But more important, perhaps, is that each year I learn, or relearn, something about the confusing contradictions young boys must deal with as they move into manhood.

The boys who are out on the patio clucking over their babies, the football players who have spent hours lovingly fashioning their cribs and cradles, are the very same boys who come up to me before class, giggling and pushing at me dog-eared copies of whatever racy, adolescent paperback novel has been making the rounds of late. "Read this, read this," they insist, the books open to pages on which "the good parts" have been underlined in red.

During the past couple of years, it's been Nick Carter novels. Possibly you aren't familiar with these, and I must admit that I have never read much more than "the good parts" of any Nick Carter novel. Apparently, though, Nick is some sort of detective or international spy or CIA operative. Nick and his fellow heroes of this particular literary genre are quite a bunch of guys. They have all sorts of thrilling adventures and narrow escapes. They are, each and every one, precision marksmen. They generally drive very fast, very expensive, very red sports cars. They are well-versed in obscure martial arts, which they regularly apply to various thugs and scoundrels of a vaguely Mafioso, Communist ilk. And of course truth, justice, the American way, and our heroes always triumph in the end. But all the intrigue and rather convoluted plots are just so much window dressing, merely something to hang "the good parts" on—for what the Nick Carter novels and the others of the genre are really about is *sex*.

Curiously enough, Nick and his literary counterparts, at least in my spotty readings, rarely seem to make the first sexual moves. Instead, it's the women who "come on" to them (a rather effective device for sidestepping the old fear-of-rejection problem).

There is nothing in the least bit shy or retiring about the ladies Nick encounters. They are a most lascivious lot. The women in these novels are forever ripping open their blouses and begging our hero to have his way with them. The hero, being a gentleman, obliges. There is a curiously Victorian coyness to the lurid detailing of these sexual exploits. It's always the hero's "manhood," his "organ," his "hardness," or his throbbing pulsating "member" that so delights the ladies and their "wet openness"— never anything so clinical, explicit, or mundane as a "penis" or a "vagina."

These sexual gymnastics often continue for several pages. As I said, Nick and his cohorts are quite a bunch of guys. Often the episodes wind to a close with the ladies expressing gratitude for the wonderful satisfaction our hero has provided and declaring their undying love for him, although as far as I've been able to determine the women and the hero rarely, if ever, meet up again.

I am not normally one to rain on anybody's parade, but when the boys in my classes ask me to read the underlined sections of books like these, I figure that they're asking for some sort of reaction, that they want to know what I think. So I tell them. I do my best to avoid being sarcastic—that clearly isn't the tack called for here. I explain that neither my sex life nor the sex life of anyone else I know on the planet proceeds along the lines described in these books. We discuss what's unreal about the sexual encounters in Nick's life and why the author chose to portray them in this light. We talk about the real-life fears and uncertainties most people have in regard to sex, about sexuality and the emotional feelings involved in being sexual with another person. From an educational point of view, we get a lot of mileage out of old Nick.

The issue I'm trying to get at here is that this culture poses some rather tricky problems for young boys trying to find their way into manhood. On the one hand, they have a tender, caring side—the side I see so clearly when they're essentially "playing dolls" with egg babies. On the other hand, they are confronted with all these thrilling and titillating images of a conquering, tough-guy male sexuality, which doesn't seem to allow much room for anybody's being at all tender or caring. It must be rather difficult to reconcile making a cradle for your egg baby with the sagas of Nick Carter. It must be very hard for a boy to sort all this out, and this undoubtedly accounts for a large portion of the adolescent male angst. Of course, what I'm talking about here isn't any great revelation. We all know that during childhood boys generally are allowed some room, given some social permission, to demonstrate or act out their tender side. And we all know that at adolescence they begin to move into the strange world of male adulthood in which, if Nick is to be believed, "real men" are not noted for their tenderness, "real men" don't cry or ever feel uncertain about who they are or what they're supposed to do, "real men" always know the right sexual moves to make, "real men" are always knowledgeable and supremely confident about sex and life in general.

To top it all off, just as they're moving from childhood into this confusing world of manhood, all these strange changes start happening to their bodies. And chances are that nobody around them seems willing to explain these changes in any but the most cursory way, if at all. In fact, the message that boys are getting is that somehow they're supposed to *know* about these things, for one of the main tenets of the male mystique is that guys, or at least "real men," automatically know everything about anything that has to do with sex.

In my classes, I show a film about male puberty entitled *Am I Normal?*, in which the central character is a boy of around twelve or thirteen years of age. He's been sprouting new hairs, getting spontaneous erections, and having wet dreams. He's trying to find out what's going on with his body and to answer the basic question that most boys this age have—that is, "Am I normal?" He goes to his father and tells him that he wants to talk about sex. Pop, who's relaxing, feet up in front of the tube watching the game, snaps off the TV and nervously asks, "What's the matter? You in trouble, or something?" The son tells him no, he just wants to know some things.

"Oh, I see," the father says, "you want to know about sex. That's terrific, son. . . . You know, my father never spoke to me about that kind of stuff." And he goes on to make an amusingly inept attempt to explain things.

"Okay, let's see now. Men have their own, uh . . . baseball bats, and girls have, uh . . . catcher's mitts. . . ."

As the father continues fumbling around with this rather awkward metaphor, the son interrupts and explains that what he really wants to know about is the change happening in his own body. The father throws up his hands and tells the son not to worry. "Men just know about these things. That's all, they just know. It'll come to you, you'll see."

But, the male mystique aside, the fact of the matter is that boys don't "just know" about these things. They have to be told. Unfortunately, they don't, as a rule, get told much of anything, either at school or in the home.

In recent years, there's been a great deal of heated public debate about the nature of sex education in our nation's schools, much of it generated by conservative parents who feel that sex education belongs in the home, and that the sexual morality implied in these classes is not up to snuff. More liberal parents have taken up the banner in response to these attacks and have loudly and ferociously defended sex-education programs. You may be a conservative or you may be a liberal. You may be on one side or the other of this debate. Being a sex-education teacher, I have my own, rather predictable, point of view on the issue. But I'm willing to concede that there are valid points to be made on each side.

In general, I think that public debate on an issue like this is a good thing. I do worry, though, that it leaves parents with the impression that there is, in fact, something to debate about, that there *are* sex-education programs throughout our nation's schools. Unfortunately, this is not the case. According to one recent survey, fewer than 10 percent of the teenagers in this country are exposed to a comprehensive sex-education program. If you've been assuming, as many parents do—especially in the wake of all this debate—that at school your boy is getting the information he needs about the sexual changes of puberty, chances are you're wrong. In most schools, sex education still consists of the kind of thing that happened when we were kids. One day, usually in the sixth grade, all the boys are mysteriously sent out to the playground for an extra "free" period, to play baseball or whatever sport is in season. The girls are herded into the auditorium and shown a film, generally produced by one of the sanitary napkin and tampon manufacturers, in which butterflies flitter through uteri and in which menstruation and the need to use these various menstrual products are explained.

The schools simply aren't doing the job we parents, for better or worse, imagine that they're doing. For the average boy, home isn't much of a source of information either. Most of the girls in my classes have been the recipients of at least one rather nervous and embarrassed "talk" from their parents (as a rule, their mothers) about menstruation, the hallmark of female puberty. But there are very few boys in my classes whose parents (either the mother or the father) have talked with them about ejaculation, the hallmark of male puberty, or about spontaneous erections, masturbation, wet dreams, or any of the other physical realities of male puberty. I'm not sure why we have decided that it's important to talk to our daughters about puberty but not so important to talk to our sons. Perhaps it has something to do with the fact that our daughter's first menstruation requires at least some sort of minimal parental response—someone's got to buy her a box of sanitary napkins or tampons and tell her how they're used and not to flush them down the toilet. When a boy ejaculates for the first time, we don't have to rush out to the store for anything, and we don't have to worry about him clogging up the plumbing. It's a lot easier to ignore our sons' "coming of age" than it is to ignore our daughters'.

Or maybe it's because our daughters bleed, and bleeding is generally recognized as a traumatic event. It's certainly true that a young girl, unprepared for her first menstrual period, may be terrified by the blood and think she's horribly sick or dying. But over the years, I've collected an equal number of stories from guys, unprepared for the possibility of wet dreams, who imagined they'd lost all control and had wet the bed, were sure they'd contracted some dread disease, or thought they were somehow being punished for masturbating.

Or perhaps it has to do with the fact that once our daughters begin to menstruate regularly, they become, for the first time, capable of getting pregnant. This fact alone seems to convince many parents that their daughters deserve some sex education. And yet, girls don't get pregnant by themselves. As my mother used to say, "It takes two to tango," although she was never talking about dancing when she said this.

Or maybe it's just the old male mystique, the belief that boys automatically know everything they need to know about sex. Few parents would actually argue that boys will magically understand what's happening to their bodies without someone telling them. But many parents have the attitude that puberty isn't really a "big deal" for boys. There's a popular idea in our culture that it's only girls who are embarrassed, anxious, and worried about the physical changes of puberty.

You couldn't prove it by me. In my sex-education classes, we play a game called Everything You Ever Wanted to Know About Sex and Puberty but Were Too Embarrassed to Ask, which involves a locked question box to which kids can anonymously submit questions. At the end of each class, I open the box, read out loud the questions that have accumulated that week, and answer them as best I can. The questions come printed in block letters (to disguise the handwriting), and the paper on which they're written has inevitably been folded about ten times into a tiny little packet. After all, this is embarrassing stuff.

Judging from the questions that come up, boys are just as curious as girls about what's happening to their bodies. For every question about menstrual periods or developing breasts, there's one about wet dreams, ejaculations, or hair growth, things like, "How much of that white stuff comes out when a guy comes?" and "When will I grow a beard and start to look like my dad?" Here's one that I got earlier this year:

> I am growing a mustash. Not a big mustash, but tiny hares. How can a boy by the age of eleven? He didn't have puberty yet.

The spelling and syntax are unusual, but the spirit behind the question isn't. This boy was worried about the fact that he was developing some fine hairs on his upper lip but he'd never "had puberty," by which he meant that he hadn't ever ejaculated. Generally, facial hair doesn't appear until the sex organs have started to develop, the boy's begun making sperm in his testicles, and he's already begun to ejaculate. But boys develop in different ways, and although it's *unusual* to develop a mustache before these other changes have begun to occur, it's certainly not *abnormal*. This boy, like most young boys, was simply looking for reassurance that what was happening to him was completely normal. It seems little enough to ask.

One reason why parents don't talk to their sons about puberty is undoubtedly simple ignorance. Most fathers didn't get much information from their own fathers. They don't exactly have a storehouse of knowledge to pass on to their sons. Although they have a general idea of what happens during puberty, having gone through it themselves, it's a rare father who can explain to his son exactly why he might have wet dreams or tell him the average age at which a boy first ejaculates. Mothers are at even more of a loss in this respect. They might feel confident enough to make a stab at telling a daughter about menstruation; after all, they've been menstruating themselves for most of their lives. But when it comes to spontaneous erections, wet dreams, and such, they're generally completely at sea.

Another factor in most parents' failure to tell their sons about the body changes of puberty is embarrassment. Sexuality is a difficult, even nigh on to impossible topic for many parents. Even those of us who feel fairly easy about discussing sex may find that there are certain areas of sexuality that we're not entirely comfortable talking over with our children. Take masturbation, for example. It's pretty difficult to discuss puberty with a boy without talking about masturbation; over 90 percent of boys masturbate during puberty. Yet masturbation is a delicate subject, and most of us are bound to feel a little embarrassed discussing it. For one thing, how in the world do you even broach the subject in the first place? What do you say? "Hi, son, been masturbating lately?"

As you may have guessed, I'm coming around to the why-I-wrote-the-book part of this introduction. The purpose of the book is, of course, to provide the basic information that young boys want and need about what's happening to their bodies as they go through puberty, information that we as parents all too often don't have available to give them. Beyond providing the basic facts, I hope that the book will help parents and sons get past the "embarrassment barrier." Ideally, I imagine parents (both the father and the mother) sitting down and reading the book with their sons. Somehow, having the facts printed on a page makes it less embarrassing—someone else is saying it, not *you*; you're just reading the information.

Of course, it's not necessary for both parents to read the book with their son. Either one parent or the other may choose to do so, or it may work better in your particular situation for you to simply give the book to your son to read on his own. You may not even have to give it to him. A number of parents who've read my book about girls and puberty, *What's Happening to My Body?: A Growing Up Guide for Mothers and Daughters*, have told me that they bought the book intending to read it with their daughters. But before they'd gotten around to giving it to them, the girls had found the book lying around the house and were already halfway through it.

Regardless of whether you read it separately or together, I hope you'll find a way to talk together about the subjects covered in the book. However, you should be prepared for the fact that, even after your son has read the book, talking it over with him may not be the easiest thing to do. If you come at it head-on by asking a direct question like, "What did you think of the book?" or "Is there anything in the book you'd like to talk about?", it's possible that you'll get a wonderfully detailed critical appraisal of the book, or a series of open, frank questions. What's more likely, though, is that you'll get something along the lines of, "It was okay," or "Naw, there's nothin' I want to know," or "I don-wanna talk about that stuff."

In my experience, it's better to take a slightly different approach. One thing that often works well is for the parent to start things off by saying something along these lines:

"Gee, when I was about your age, I _____."
(Fill in the blank: "noticed my first hairs," "had my first wet dream," "ejaculated for the first time," or whatever.)
"I felt really _____."
("Nervous," "excited," "proud," "embarrassed," "afraid," or whatever.)
"In fact, what happened to me was that I _____
_____." (Again, fill in the blank with a story about something from your own adolescence, the more embarrassing or stupid the story, the better.)

By using this approach, you make it easier for your kid to open up. By virtue of whatever embarrassing, dumb story you've told about yourself, you've let your kid know that it's okay to be uncertain and less than all-knowingly perfect about the whole business. At least the kids in my class always seem to open up when I tell them about things like:

- The time I got my menstrual period without knowing it and walked around school half the day with a big red blotch on my skirt before anyone told me, and how after that I was sure I could never face going back to school again in my whole life.
- Or the time I bet my best friend, Georgia, my entire allowance that the way people had babies was: the man kissed the woman; a seed from his belly came up his throat, went into her mouth and down her throat, landing in her belly;

and nine months later, a baby came out of her belly button. I lost my entire allowance to Georgia.

- Or the time my brother ran for class president and had to give a speech in the auditorium in front of everyone in the whole school, and got a spontaneous erection and didn't know if everyone was laughing at the jokes in his speech or the fact that he had a hard-on.

You get the idea.

Here's another pearl of wisdom: avoid having one all-purposeful "talk." It won't fill the bill, no matter how hard you try. It's also better to approach things casually, bringing up the topic from time to time when it seems natural to do so. When I was beginning puberty, my mother sat me down one day to have the Talk. I'm sure she must have explained things in a fairly comprehensible way. All I recall, though, was my mother being horribly nervous and embarrassed and saying a lot of stuff about blood and babies. Then she said something about how when it happened to me, I could come and get some napkins out of the bottom drawer of her bedroom dresser. I remember wondering why in the world she'd be keeping napkins in the bottom drawer of her dresser instead of the top drawer of the kitchen cabinet, which was where napkins were normally kept in our house. But my mother was acting so weird that it just didn't seem like the kind of question to ask at the time. In my experience, a more casual, spur-of-the-moment approach to talking to your child about puberty works better.

Yet another piece of advice: if talking about puberty and sexuality is difficult or embarrassing for you, say so. There's nothing wrong with telling your child, "This is really embarrassing for me. . .," or "My parents never talked to me about this stuff, so I feel kind of weird trying to talk to you. . .," or whatever. Your child is going to pick up on your embarrassment anyway from your tone of voice, your body language, or any one of the other ways we have of communicating what we're really feeling. By trying to pretend you're not uncomfortable, you'll only succeed in confusing your child. Once you've admitted your feelings, you've cleared the air. Your child may adopt a maddeningly smug attitude or be patronizingly sympathetic about your embarrassment, but in the end this is preferable to having him think that there is something weird about the topic itself, that it's not quite right to talk about it.

At this point I must say something about the question that parents most often ask: At what age should you tell your kids about these things? Conventional wisdom holds that you wait until the kids start asking questions. Like many bits of conventional wisdom, this strikes me as a piece of utter nonsense. We don't wait until our kids ask before we teach them how to cross the street safely. Or, if we're religious people, we don't wait until they ask about God before we give them religious instruction. Nor should we wait until they ask before we talk to them about puberty and sex. For one thing, we might end up waiting forever. Kids, having been the recipients of endless unsolicited parental guidance about virtually everything else in their lives, are not very likely to come asking questions about the one area we've been so studiously avoiding. The very fact of our silence on the topic of sexuality sends our kids the message that this is something that it's not okay to talk about.

To my mind, sex education should begin when our children are toddlers. This is not to suggest that you should provide your three-year-old with a sex manual describing sixty-eight different positions for intercourse, or bog down young minds with a detailed explanation of the hormones that initiate and regulate puberty. But once your child reaches the bedtime-story stage, it seems altogether appropriate to introduce the topics of conception, birth, sexuality, and puberty by means of any of the many fine children's picture books that deal with these topics. (Some of my favorites are listed in For Further Reading at the back of this book.)

The book you have here was designed for boys in the nine- to fifteen-year-old group, although it may be appropriate for younger or older boys as well. If sex and related topics are subjects you've been discussing with your child all along, I think you'll find this book is a good bridge between the picture books for younger kids and the publications available for older teens (again, some of my favorite books for older teens are listed in For Further Reading). If this book is your first foray into the sex education of your child, I think that you'll find it an excellent starting place.

I hope the book is one that you'll reread with your son time and again as he's growing older, or that you'll keep around the house so that he can go back to it. What a child of eight or nine takes away from this book will be different from what a boy of thirteen or fourteen does. For example, Chapter 5 deals with spontaneous erections, ejaculations, wet dreams, and masturbation. In my experience, boys of nine or ten are quite curious about these topics, even though most don't actually have their first wet dreams and ejaculations until they are thirteen, fourteen, or older. In fact, younger boys are often more open and easy about discussing these topics than they will be a few years later, when they are experiencing them. At nine or ten, a boy may read Chapter 5 and take away a certain understanding; but at age thirteen or fourteen, when these things are much more real and immediate, the information will be meaningful in different ways. It's important that a boy be prepared for the pubertal changes described in the first five chapters of this book before they happen, but it's also important that he be able to go back and reread the information after these changes have started to take place in his own body.

Chapter 6 deals with girls and puberty. I think it's a good idea for younger boys to have this kind of information. But it will be seen in a different light and taken in by the boy in a more meaningful way once his female classmates have actually begun to go through these changes. So here again, it's important that your boy have this information to go back to as he grows older.

I don't pretend to cover everything here that you'll need to discuss with your child as he moves through puberty and adolescence. What book could? This is only a beginning. It doesn't go into detail about topics like birth control, venereal disease, rape, incest, abortion, sexuality, or making decisions about sex. However, it does touch upon these subjects. Chapter 7 is a question-and-answer chapter in which I address the questions kids in my sex-education classes most frequently ask (those that I haven't already addressed in the first six chapters); these sorts of topics are discussed briefly there, along with references to other books and sources of information about them.

As a parent, you may find that you have some concerns about some of the material covered in this book. Some of the topics, especially those touched upon in Chapter 7, are very controversial. When controversial questions come up in class, I try to present the various points of view and explain why people have them. I think I do a pretty good job of being objective. But sometimes my own point of view comes through. For instance, when discussing masturbation, I explain that some people feel it is wrong or sinful and not at all a good thing to do, and I talk about why they feel that way. But the truth of the matter is that I feel very strongly that masturbation is a perfectly fine, perfectly normal thing to do, and I'm sure that this comes through in what I've written. You may find that your opinions on masturbation or some of the other topics covered in this book are different from mine, but this doesn't mean you have to "throw the baby out with the bath water," as the expression goes. Instead, you can use these differences as an opportunity to explain and elucidate your own attitudes and values to your child.

Another concern you may have is that this book covers topics that you don't want your child to know about. I'm thinking here of birth control. Many parents don't want their children to have information about birth control for fear that this will lead them to become sexually active. I disagree with this point of view entirely. I think that the studies done on this issue make it clear that giving teenagers informaion on birth control *does not* make it more likely that they'll have sexual intercourse. However, keep in mind that the information on birth control in this book is not how-to information. It is merely a brief description of the various methods of contraception, and it is general enough so that I don't think it will pose much of a problem even for those parents who have a more conservative attitude on the subject.

Yet another concern that you may have is that your child may be too young for some of the information in this book. This won't be a problem with Chapters 1 through 6, but in Chapter 7, for instance, topics like oral-genital sex come up. Questions about this topic do get asked in the "Everything You Wanted to Know . . ." question box I use in my classes. Of course, kids don't use the term oral-genital sex when they ask about it—they want to know what the slang words they've heard for it mean. So, in class and here in this book, I've provided a brief discussion of the topic. (And I do mean brief; please don't get the idea that there's any titillatingly detailed discussion of the topic either in my classes or in this book.)

It's only natural for us to wonder if it's really necessary to tell our nine- or ten- or twelve-year-olds, or even our older children, about some of the topics covered in Chapter 7. Aren't they a bit young? Do they really need to know about these sorts of things? And the answer is, Of course, they don't need to know about them. But the fact of the matter is that they probably already do, or they will be hearing about them before much longer. For better or for worse, our children are subjected to a barrage of information on a variety of topics about which most of us were blissfully ignorant when we were their ages. In some cases, I think it is for the better. For example, I think it's a good thing that topics like incest are being discussed openly. Unpleasant as it is to think about, incest does happen, to millions of kids, and nothing can be done to stop it unless we talk about it openly. But in other cases, you may feel that a subject like oral-genital sex is not one you'd choose, of your accord, to bring up with a ten- or eleven-year-old. It certainly doesn't fall into the need-to-know category, at least not for kids just going through puberty.

Yet, as I said, today's children learn about these things long before they have a need to know about them. The topic came up in class one of the first years I was teaching because the kids had gone on an outing to a nearby park. A group of boys, some of the older as well as younger ones, had gone to the public bathroom and had discovered, taped to the wall of one of the stalls, a series of pictures from a porno magazine of a couple engaging in this activity. The whole incident became a *very big deal* at school and was soon passed along the grapevine, whispered from child to child, until almost all the kids in school had gotten wind of it.

As a teacher, it seemed to me that it was better to talk openly about the incident in class than to simply ignore it. The reaction of most kids was, "Ugh! Why would anyone even want to do that?" I was able to explain that some adults find this kind of lovemaking a special way of giving each other sexual pleasure and of being close. I talked about how there was nothing "dirty" about it from a sanitary point of view. I explained that some people feel this kind of lovemaking is sinful or morally wrong, while others feel it's perfectly okay. And, what's perhaps most important, I was able to let the kids know that oral-genital sex isn't something you *have* to do when you grow up and start having sex with another person. Like everything else about sex, it is something you can either decide to do or decide not to do, depending on how you personally feel about it. This is important, for kids hearing or learning about things like this can get the mistaken idea that they're things you have to do, and this can make them very uncertain and fearful about sex in general.

Maybe you feel it would be better if we could turn back the clock and raise our children in a world where at least they'd be less likely to come across pornographic pictures taped to the wall of a public bathroom; or perhaps you feel that the increased exposure to sexual information is not altogether a bad thing. Regardless of how you feel, as parents we must recognize that our kids are exposed to a great deal more sexual information than most of us were at their age. My personal philosophy is to take the bull by the horns and to discuss these kinds of things with our children. In some cases, this may mean that we bring up topics that they haven't yet heard about from their friends or gleaned from the media. Even if it is new information when your child is nine years old, though, I'd be willing to bet that it's something he'll have heard about before he's thirteen or fourteen. I think it is far better that they get information from us than from porno magazines or from the talk they share with their friends.

You may feel that you'd rather wait until your child is older to broach some of the topics discussed in Chapter 7. If so, please follow your own instincts on this. Decide what portions of Chapter 7 you think are appropriate and which, if any, you find inappropriate. Then simply read the book to your child, skipping over any portions you don't feel comfortable with.

Regardless of how you decide to deal with the topics of puberty and sexuality or how you decide to use this book, I hope that it will help you and your child to gain a greater understanding of the process of puberty and that it will bring the two of you closer together.

CHAPTER 1

Puberty

It was great. I remember thinking, "I'm not just a kid any-more!" I loved it!

John, age 26

It was weird. I was tired all the time and sleeping a whole lot. I wasn't really sure what was happening to me.

Bill, age 19

People make it sound like it's this big dramatic thing that all of a sudden happens one day. It's not like that. It's not like some guy pops up and says, "Hey, kid, this is it. Now it's going to happen to you."

Jackson, age 33

It seemed like I woke up one day and everything had changed. I was a different person in a different body.

Sam, age 35

Even though they had very different things to say about it, all these men are talking about the same thing

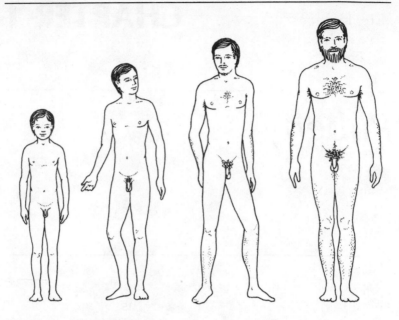

Illustration 1. Male puberty changes. As boys go through puberty, they get taller, their shoulders get wider, their bodies more muscular, their genital organs develop, and they begin to grow hair on their genitals, underarms, faces, chests, arms and legs.

—puberty.* Puberty is a time in people's lives when their bodies are changing from children's bodies into adults' bodies. As you can see from Illustration 1, a boy's body changes quite a bit as he goes through puberty. For one thing, he gets taller. Of course, we grow taller all through childhood. But during puberty, a boy grows taller at a faster rate than he ever will again in his

---

* *puberty* (PEW-bur-tee)   The word puberty is pronounced with the accent on the first part of the word, PEW. You say this part of the word loudest, with the most emphasis. Throughout this book, there are a number of words that you may not have heard before. Whenever we use one of these words for the first time, we have included a pronunciation guide like this at the bottom of the page.

life. During this growth spurt, he may gain as many as five inches in one year.

The general shape of his body changes too, so that his shoulders become broader and his hips seem narrower in comparison. His muscles develop and his body strength increases. His whole body begins to look more "manly." Hair grows in places where it never grew before—around his penis, under his arms, and on his face. His penis and his scrotum, the sac of skin just beneath his penis, get bigger. At the same time that these changes are happening on the outside of his body, other changes are taking place on the inside of his body.

For some boys, these changes happen so fast that they seem to take place overnight. But they don't really happen that quickly. Puberty happens slowly and gradually, over a period of months or years. These changes may start when a boy is as young as ten. Or they may not happen until he is fifteen. Regardless of when they start for you, you'll probably have a lot of questions about what is happening to your body. We hope this book will answer at least some of those questions.

"We" are my friend Dane and I. The two of us worked together to make this book. About a year before I wrote this book, my daughter, Area, and I wrote another book, a lot like this one, about how puberty happens in girls' bodies. (It's called *What's Happening to my Body?: A Growing Up Guide for Mothers and Daughters*.) Even though I'm a medical writer and teach classes about puberty and know a lot of scientific facts about puberty, I thought it would be a good idea

penis (PEE-niss)
scrotum (SKRO-tum)

to get my daughter's help in writing the girl's book. She was going through puberty herself at the time. Of course, I had been through puberty too, but it was a long time ago. I was thirty-six when Area and I wrote the girl's book, and to tell you the truth, I wasn't really sure I could think back across all those years and remember the kinds of feelings and questions I had back then. I figured Area could give me the kid's point of view on things. So I talked her into writing the girl's book with me, and I guess we did a pretty good job because Esther Margolis, the woman who published the girl's book, said, "Why don't you do a book about boys and puberty?"

I thought that sounded like a good idea, but once again, I wanted to get the kid's point of view. It seemed especially important for this book because I'm a woman, and I don't have firsthand knowledge of how puberty happens in a boy's body. The trouble was that I don't have a son. So I decided to find a boy that I knew really well and who felt comfortable enough with me and with himself to work on a book like this. That's when I thought of Dane. Dane's mom, Katie, and I have been good friends for years and years, and I've known Dane ever since he barely came up to my knees. (He's way past my knees now. In fact, he's fifteen and six feet tall and I have to stick my nose up in the air when I want to talk to him.)

Dane thought the idea of doing this book sounded good too, so he agreed to provide the kid's point of view. He read over the various parts of the book and told me when I'd written something really dumb or when I'd forgotten to explain something or when what I'd said was confusing or unclear. And we both talked to lots of men and boys to find out what happened to *them* during puberty, how they felt about it, and what kinds of questions and concerns they had at the time. You'll hear their voices throughout this book. Some of the quotes we've used are from kids in my classes.* During the school year, I teach a class in puberty at Sequoyah School in Pasadena, California. The kids in my classes and the men and boys Dane and I talked to had a lot of questions and a lot of things to say about puberty. So, in a sense, they too helped write this book.

Way back when I first started teaching classes about puberty, I decided that the best way to begin was to talk about how babies are made, because the changes that happen in our bodies during puberty happen because we are getting ready for a time when we may decide to make babies.

I didn't think I'd have any big problems in teaching the class. "Nothing to it," I told myself. "I'll just go on in there and start by talking to the kids about how babies are made. Probably I'll have to draw some pictures on the blackboard to help explain things, and maybe I don't draw really well, but we'll manage."

"No problem," I told myself.

Boy, was I wrong. I'd hardly even opened my mouth before everyone, or almost everyone, in the class started acting crazy. Kids were giggling and nudging one another and getting all red in the face. One boy even fell off his chair. People were acting all sorts of strange ways because, in order to talk about how babies are made, I had to talk about *sex*, and sex, as you may have noticed, is a *very big deal*. Kids—and, in fact, people of all ages—often act embarrassed, giggly, or secretive when the topic of sex comes up.

* We changed the names of the boys and men we quoted in this book in order not to embarrass them after they'd been generous enough to share their feelings and thoughts about puberty with us.

Even the word itself is confusing because *sex* can mean so many different things and is used in so many different ways. In the simplest meaning of the word, *sex* refers to the different kinds of bodies that men and women have. There are a lot of differences between male and female bodies, but one of the most obvious is that a male has a penis and a scrotum, and a female has a vulva and a vagina. These body parts, or organs (*organ* is another word for body part), are called *sex organs*. People belong to either the male sex or the female sex, depending on which type of sex organs they have.

The word *sex* is also used in other ways. We may say that two people are "having sex." Having sex, or having *sexual intercourse*, involves a man putting his penis into a woman's vagina. Or we may say that two people are "being sexual with each other," which means that they are having sexual intercourse or that they are holding, touching, or caressing each other's sexual organs. We may say that we are "feeling sexual," which means that we are having feelings or thoughts about our sexual organs, about being sexual with another person, or about having sexual intercourse.

Our sex organs are very private parts of our bodies. We usually keep them covered up, and we don't talk about them in public very often. Having sex, being sexual with someone, or having sexual feelings are also private matters that don't get talked about very often. I suppose that if I'd had half a brain in my head, I would have realized that coming into a classroom and talking about sex and penises and vaginas and making

vulva (VUL-va)
vagina (vah-JIE-nah)
intercourse (IN-ter-korse)

babies and all that stuff that people don't usually talk about was going to cause a big commotion.

After that first class, though, I caught on. I decided that if we were going to get all silly and giggly when we talked about these things in class, we might as well get *really* silly and giggly. So now I start the first class of the year by giving everyone photocopies of the two drawings you see in Illustration 2 and red and blue colored pencils that we use to color the drawings.

THE SEX ORGANS

Illustration 2 shows the female and male sex organs, also called the *genitals* or *genital organs*. Everyone has sex organs on both the inside and outside of the body, and they change as we go through puberty. These pictures show how the sex organs on the outside of the body look in grown men and women.

Nowadays, I start my puberty classes by holding up the picture of the male sex organs. I explain to the class that the sex organs on the outside of a man's body have two main parts and that the scientific names for these parts are the *penis* and the *scrotum*. When I pass out the drawings and start talking about the penis and the scrotum, the kids in my class still giggle like mad, nudge one another, or fall off their chairs in embarrassment, but I don't pay much attention to all of this. I simply say, "Okay, the penis itself also has two parts: the *shaft* and the *glans*. Find the shaft of the penis on your drawing and color it with blue and red stripes." Some kids keep giggling and some get very serious about the coloring, but they all start coloring. Why don't you color

genitals (JEN-a-tulls)
glans (GLANZ)

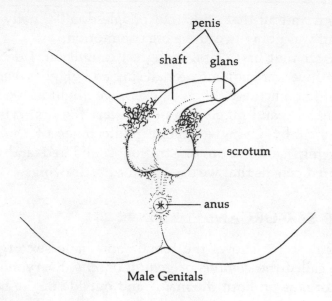

Male Genitals

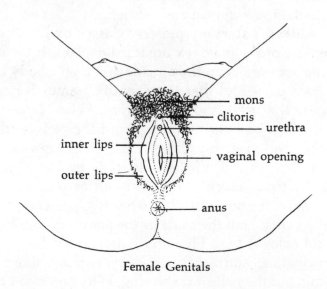

Female Genitals

Illustration 2. Male and female genitals

the shaft in, too. (Unless, of course, this book belongs to someone else or to a library. One of the people we admire most in the world is a wonderful lady named Lou Ann Sobieski. She's a librarian, and Dane and I would be in *very hot water* if Lou Ann thought we were telling people to color on library books.)

The glans, or head, of the penis has a ridge of skin around the lower part called the *corona*, and after the class has colored the shaft, I tell them to color the corona red. There's usually a bit less giggling by now as they start coloring the corona, because it's smaller and they have to pay more attention to what they are doing. Next, we color in the glans itself. I usually recommend blue, but color it any way you want, just as long as it's colored differently from the other parts so that it will stand out clearly. Then, we color in the small opening in the center of the glans called the *urinary opening*. This is the opening through which urine (pee) leaves the body.

Next comes the scrotum. "Red and blue polka dots for the scrotum," I tell my class. By this time, the picture is beginning to look rather silly, and the giggling has turned to outright laughter.

The scrotum is a loose bag of skin that lies beneath the penis. Another name for the scrotum is the scrotal sac. Inside the scrotum are two egg-shaped organs called *testes* or *testicles*. You can't see them in these pictures, but I like to mention them at this point because they have a lot to do with making babies. (We'll talk more about them in the following pages.)

corona (ko-RO-na)
urinary (YUR-in-airee)
urine (YUR-in)
testes (TES-teez)
testicles (TES-ti-kuls)

I also explain that the curly hairs they see growing around the genitals have a special name. These hairs are called *pubic hairs*.

Finally, we come to the *anus*. The anus is the opening through which feces or bowel movements leave our bodies. It's not really a sex organ, but because it is located in the genital area, I like to mention it.

By the time we've colored in the different parts, I've said the word *penis* in front of the class about twenty-eight times, so everyone gets used to my saying this word that usually doesn't get said out loud in classrooms (or anywhere else for that matter), and they no longer have to get all crazy and giggly each time I use it. Besides that, the pictures look so funny that everyone gets to laughing out loud, and that makes it easier for all of us to deal with the nervousness that most of us feel when we talk about sex organs.

I also have another reason for getting the kids in my class to color in these drawings: I think it helps them to learn the names of these organs. If you just look at the drawing and see that this part is labeled the *penis* and that part the *scrotum*, it's all kind of jumbled and doesn't stick in your mind. But if you spend a few moments coloring them in, you have to pay attention and you'll remember better. These are important parts of the body, so it's worth the effort. If this book isn't yours and you can't color in it, try making a tracing of these drawings and coloring on the tracing.

While we're going through the business of coloring the drawings, we also talk about slang words. As you know, people don't always use the scientific names for

pubic (PEW-bic)
anus (AY-nus)
feces (FEE-sees)
bowel (BOW-ul)

these body parts. Mostly they use slang words. I've found that if we don't talk about these words right out loud in class, kids are always leaning over and whispering them to one another and giggling madly and acting crazy again. So while we're coloring our drawings, all of the kids yell out the slang words they've heard for penis, scrotum, and testicles and I make a list of them on the blackboard. Here are some of the words that we've come up with:

SLANG WORDS FOR THE PENIS, SCROTUM,
AND TESTICLES

PENIS			*SCROTUM AND TESTICLES*	
cock	peter	tool	balls	cujones
dick	rod	frankfurter	nuts	things
prick	dingus	thing	eggs	bangers
schlong	dork	banger	rocks	hangers
wee-wee	meat	dinky	jewels	stones
wanger	pisser	penie	cubes	seeds
pecker	hot dog	weenie	sac	bag
wang	weiner	dong		

As I explain to the kids in my class, I personally don't object to using slang words to refer to sex organs. In fact, I think that they are sometimes easier to use and they make people more comfortable about talking about these body parts. But some people do object to these slang words, and they may get upset if they hear you using them. You may or may not care about upsetting people in this way, but you should at least be aware that there are people who find slang words offensive.

Next, I usually show my class a picture like the one in Illustration 3 and explain about circumcision.

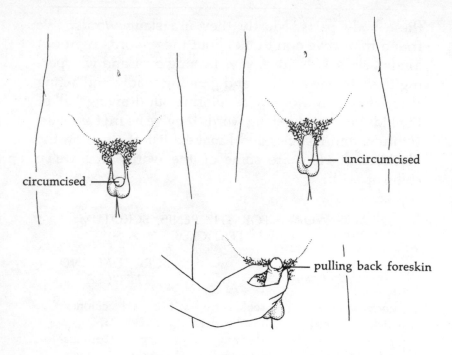

circumcised

uncircumcised

pulling back foreskin

Illustration 3. Circumcision

Circumcision is an operation in which the doctor cuts away a fold of skin called the *foreskin* from around the top of the penis. The foreskin covers the glans of the penis, but it can be pulled down the shaft, as shown in Illustration 3. In this country, most circumcisions are done when babies are two or three days old. The foreskin is pulled up over the top of the penis and a special instrument is used to cut the foreskin away. Not all parents choose to have their babies circumcised. If you have not been circumcised, it is important that you pull the foreskin back and clean under it whenever you bathe or shower, because a secretion called smegma

circumcision (sir-cum-SISH-un)
circumcised (sir-cum-SIZED)
smegma (SMEG-ma)

collects under the foreskin and can cause an unpleasant odor or irritation.

One of the first questions that the kids in my class ask when I talk about this subject is, Why do people have their babies circumcised? Sometimes it is done for religious reasons. It is a custom in the Jewish and Muslim religions for parents to circumcise their boys. Until recently, most boys in this country were circumcised even if their parents were not Jewish or Muslim. Doctors encouraged circumcision because it makes it easier to clean the penis, because they felt the foreskin could trap germs and the boy could be more likely to get an infection, and because it was thought that uncircumcised men were more likely to get cancer of the penis. But as long as a boy pulls the foreskin back and cleans the glans of the penis regularly, he isn't any more likely to get infections than someone who has been circumcised. Moreover, doctors are no longer certain that being circumcised really has anything to do with how likely it is that a man will get cancer of the penis. Besides, cancer of the penis is a rare disease. (Boys, by the way, *never* get cancer of the penis. It only happens to men, usually only to men over the age of fifty.) Because of all this, many doctors and parents are wondering whether it is really worth it to put a newborn baby through the pain and discomfort of circumcision. In the past ten years or so, more and more parents have been deciding not to have their male babies circumcised.

As we said, the operation is usually done when the baby is two or three days old. Occasionally, though, a boy or man who wasn't circumcised at birth may decide to have the operation done later on. Often this is because his foreskin is too tight or is stuck to the head of the penis and cannot be fully rolled down the shaft. This can cause swelling and pain, and circumcision is often the best solution. But these problems are very rare. It is unusual for an older boy or man to have the circumcision operation. If you haven't been circumcised at birth, you probably never will be.

The only difference between circumcised and uncircumcised males is that circumcised males don't have a foreskin. Otherwise, their penis looks, feels, and works the same way.

When we have finished coloring the male sex organs, we move on to the female sex organs shown in Illustration 2. The genital organs on the outside of a woman's body are sometimes referred to as the *vulva*. The vulva has many parts. We usually start at the top with the fleshy mound called the *mons*, which, in grown women, is covered with crisp, curly pubic hairs. We color the mons with blue polka dots. Then, we move toward the bottom of the mons where it divides into two folds or flaps of skin called the *outer lips*. Try coloring these with red stripes. In between the outer lips lie the *inner lips*—blue stripes for the inner lips. The inner lips join together at the top, and there is a small, bud-shaped organ called the *clitoris*. Color it red. Just down from the clitoris is the woman's urinary opening, through which urine leaves the body. Color it blue. Below the urinary opening is another opening called the *vaginal opening*. It leads into a hollow pouch or cavity inside the body called the *vagina*. Use your imagination—color it red, blue, striped, polka-dot, or whatever.

You may have heard people use the word *vagina* to refer to the vulva. Actually, the vagina is *inside* the body. The vulva, which includes the lips, the clitoris, and the urinary and vaginal openings, is on the outside

mons (MONZ)
clitoris (KLIT-or-iss)
vaginal (VAH-jin-ul)

of the body. It is not really correct to mix these terms up, but people do it all the time.

Finally, we come to the *anus*. Color it as well.

While we're coloring in the female genitals, we also make a list of slang words used to refer to these parts of a woman's body.

SLANG WORDS FOR THE CLITORIS,
VULVA, AND VAGINA

CLITORIS	*VULVA AND VAGINA*		
clit	cunt	box	snatch
bud	pussy	beaver	poontang
pea	muff	honeypot	pudie
man in the boat	stuff	hole	slit

By the time we've finished coloring both these pictures, everyone has giggled off a good deal of embarrassment. The kids have also gotten a pretty good idea of where these body parts are, which makes it a lot easier to understand how a man and a woman make babies.

SEXUAL INTERCOURSE

In order to make a baby, a man and a woman must have sexual intercourse. When I tell the kids in my class about this, they usually have two questions. One thing they want to know is how a man's penis could get into a woman's vagina. I explain that sometimes the penis gets stiff and hard and stands out from the body, as shown in Illustration 4. This is called an *erection*, and it can happen when a male is feeling sexual or is having sex with someone, and at other times too. The inside of the

erection (e-REK-shun)

penis is made up of spongy tissue. When a male is having an erection, special blood passageways in this spongy tissue fill up with blood, which makes the penis get bigger and harder and stand out from the body. Some people call an erection a "boner" or a "hard-on" because the penis feels so stiff and hard. It's almost as if there really is a bone in there. But there isn't any bone, just blood-filled, spongy tissue.

While it is erect, the penis can slide right into the vaginal opening. The vaginal opening isn't very large, but it's very elastic and stretchy, so the erect penis can easily fit in there.

In addition to wanting to know *how*, some of the kids in our classes want to know *why* in the world anyone would want to do this.

A man and a woman have sexual intercourse for all sorts of reasons. It is a special way of being close with

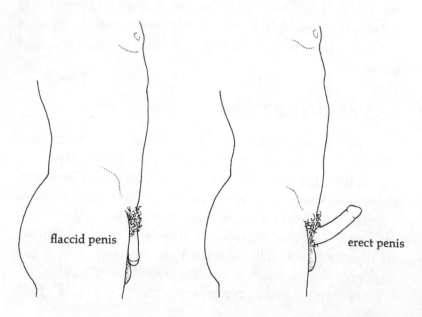

flaccid penis   erect penis

Illustration 4. Erection

another person. It also feels good, which some of the kids in my class find hard to believe. But the sex organs have many nerve endings. If these parts of our bodies are stroked or rubbed in the right ways, the nerve endings send messages to pleasure centers in our brains, and we get pleasurable feelings all over our bodies. People also have sexual intercourse because they want to have a baby, but babies don't start to grow every time a man and a woman have intercourse, just sometimes.

MAKING BABIES

In order to make a baby, two things are needed: an *ovum* from a woman's body and a *sperm* from a man's body. You may have heard adults talking about an ovum and calling it "a woman's egg" or talking about a sperm and calling it "a man's seed." When many of the kids in my classes hear the word *egg*, they think about the kind of eggs that chickens lay and that we buy at grocery stores to scramble up for breakfast. When they hear the word *seed*, they think about the things we plant in the ground in order to grow flowers or vegetables. But the ovum and the sperm are not like these kinds of eggs and seeds. For one thing, an ovum is much smaller than the eggs we cook up for breakfast—in fact, it is much smaller than the smallest dot you could make with the tip of even the sharpest pencil point. And a sperm is even smaller than an ovum.

I think the best way to think of a sperm and an ovum is to think of each of them as being half of a seed. When these two halves of a seed come together, a human baby begins to grow.

ovum (OH-vum)
sperm (SPURM)

Sperm are made in the testicles, the two egg-shaped organs inside the scrotum. Sometimes, when a man and a woman are having sexual intercourse, and the man's penis is inside the woman's vagina, a man ejaculates. When a man ejaculates, the muscles of the penis contract, and the sperm are pumped out of the testicles, through a hollow tube in the center of the penis, and out the opening in the center of the glans, as shown in Illustration 5. A teaspoon of a creamy fluid, full of millions of tiny, microscopic sperm, comes out of the penis. This liquid is called ejaculate, or in slang terms "come" or "jism."

After the sperm leave the penis, they start swimming up toward the top of the vagina. They pass through a tiny opening at the top of the vagina that leads into an organ called the *uterus* (see Illustration 6). The uterus is a hollow organ, and, in a grown woman, it is only about the size of a clenched fist. But the thick muscular walls of the uterus are quite elastic, and, like a balloon, the uterus can expand to many times its size. The uterus has to be able to expand like this because it is here, inside a woman's uterus, that a baby grows.

Some of the sperm swim up to the top of the uterus and into one of two little tubes or tunnels called the *fallopian tubes*. Not all the sperm make it this far. Some drift back down to the uterus and out into the vagina, where they join other sperm that never made it out of the vagina. These sperm and the rest of the creamy, white liquid dribble back down the vagina and out of the woman's body.

Women, too, make seeds in their bodies. When we

ejaculates (e-JACK-you-lates)
ejaculate (e-JACK-you-lat)
uterus (YOU-ter-us)
fallopian (fuh-LOPE-e-an)

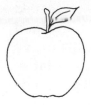 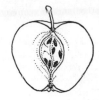 If you cut an apple in half, you would be able to see the seeds and core on the inside of the apple. This drawing, which shows the inside of an apple, is called a cross section.

The drawing below is also a cross section. It shows the inside of the penis and scrotum.

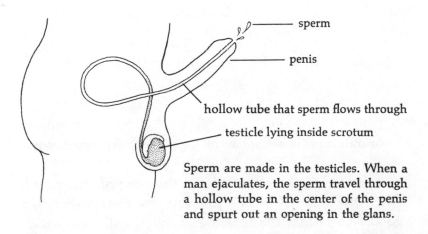

sperm

penis

hollow tube that sperm flows through

testicle lying inside scrotum

Sperm are made in the testicles. When a man ejaculates, the sperm travel through a hollow tube in the center of the penis and spurt out an opening in the glans.

Illustration 5. Ejaculation

are talking about just one of these seeds, we use the word *ovum*. When we are talking about more than one, we use the word *ova*. The ova ripen inside two little organs called *ovaries*. In a grown woman, the ovaries produce a ripe seed about once a month. When this seed is ripe, it leaves the ovary and travels down the fallopian tube toward the uterus. If a woman and man

ova (OH-vah)
ovaries (OH-vah-reez)

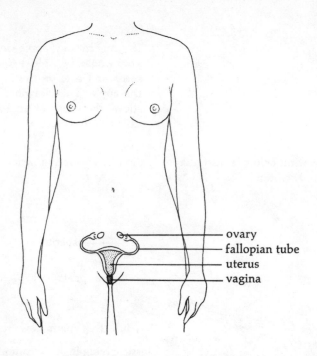

ovary
fallopian tube
uterus
vagina

Illustration 6. The sex organs on the inside of the female body

have sexual intercourse around the time of the month when the ripe ovum has just left the ovary, there's a good chance that the sperm and ovum will meet inside the tube. When a sperm and ovum meet, the sperm penetrates the outer shell of the ovum and moves inside it. This joining together of the ovum and the sperm is called fertilization, and when a sperm has penetrated an ovum, we say that the ovum has been fertilized.

Most of the time, the ovum travels through the fallopian tube without meeting up with a sperm, and the tiny ovum just disintegrates. But if the ovum has been fertilized, it doesn't disintegrate. Instead, the fertilized seed plants itself on one of the inside walls of the uterus, and over the next nine months, it grows into a

fertilization (FUR-till-ih-zay-shun)

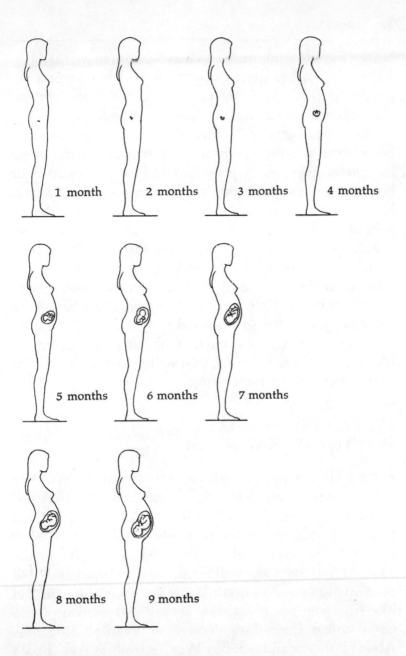

Illustration 7. Stages of pregnancy. A fertilized ovum plants itself on the inside wall of the uterus, and over the next nine months, it develops into a baby.

baby (see Illustration 7). When a woman is ready to have a baby, her uterus opens up and her vagina expands so that the baby can move from the uterus, through the vagina, and out into the world.

During puberty, girls make their first ripe ova and boys begin making sperm in their testicles. Girls begin to develop breasts, to grow hair in new places on their bodies, and to go through other important changes, both on the inside and outside of their bodies. As we said at the beginning of this chapter, boys' bodies also change, both on the inside and on the outside, as they go through puberty. In the following chapters, we will talk about the changes that take place in a boy's body during puberty. (We have also included a chapter on the changes that a girl goes through during puberty, because most boys are curious about girls.) If you're like the kids in my classes, you will probably have a lot of questions about these things.

EVERYTHING YOU EVER WANTED TO KNOW . . .

It isn't always easy to ask certain questions. We may feel too embarrassed to ask, or we may feel that our questions are too dumb. Sometimes we have questions that we would really like to know the answers to, but we think that everyone else already knows. We may be worried that everyone will think we are stupid and "out of it" if we show we don't know by asking. If you feel like this, you are not alone. In my classes, we play a game called Everything You Ever Wanted to Know About Puberty and Sex but Were Afraid to Ask. I pass out slips of paper at the beginning of each class so that the kids can write down their questions and put them in a special question box. They don't have to sign their names to the questions. I am the only one who gets to see them, so nobody can look at the handwriting and figure out who wrote the question. I also leave the locked question box and some slips of paper somewhere in the classroom so that kids can write down questions whenever one crosses their mind. At the end of each class, I take the questions out of the box, read them out loud, and answer them the best I can.

Here are some of the many kinds of questions that have come up in our question box:

"When will I grow a beard and start to look like my dad?"

"How much of that white stuff comes out of a man's penis when he ejaculates?"

"Why do you sometimes get a hard-on when you're not even thinking about sex?"

"Is there something wrong if you have one testicle lower than the other?"

"Why do you have to wear a jockstrap?"

"What's the largest penis measurement in the world? Can a penis be too small? Will it get bigger when I get older?"

"Which way should your penis curve when it's hard?"

"How come people get pimples when they're going through puberty?"

"What is a wet dream?"

"Can a boy grow breasts?"

"Exactly what does 'jacking off' or 'playing with yourself' mean, and is it okay to do it?"

"I have little white bumps on my penis. Does that mean I have some kind of disease?"

"How do twins and triplets happen? Do they come out at the same time?"

"I have a pain in my penis and some white stuff that looks like milk has been coming out. What's wrong?"

"How old should a person be before they have sex?"

"How long can sperm live?"

"If you ejaculate too often, can this hurt you? Will you run out of sperm?"

"Is it true that girls bleed once a month after they go through puberty?"

In the following pages, we will answer these and other questions that have come up in the question box or that were asked by the boys and men we talked to about puberty. You may find that you have questions that are not answered by this book. If so, perhaps your dad or mom, the school nurse, one of your teachers, or another adult you know can help you find answers to your questions. Friends your own age may be able to answer your questions, but a lot of kids find that the answers they get from other kids are not always right. It is usually better to ask an adult you know and feel comfortable talking to. Or you could write to us. We would love to hear about any questions or concerns you may have or about things you liked or didn't like about this book. Your envelope should be addressed like this:

Lynda Madaras and Dane Saavedra
Newmarket Press
3 East 48th Street
New York, New York 10017

Be sure to include your name and address if you want us to write back to you.

USING THIS BOOK

You may want to read this book with your parents, with a friend, or all by yourself. You may want to read it straight through from beginning to end, or you may want to jump around, reading a chapter here and there, depending on what you are most curious about. However you decide to go about using this book, we hope that you will enjoy it and that you will learn as much from reading it as we did from writing it.

CHAPTER 2

The Stages of Puberty

Growing vegetables is one of my hobbies. Three or four mornings a week, I'm out there in my garden pulling up weeds or planting things or yelling at the birds, which are always eating up my peas. I like to pretend that my hobby is a very sensible one and that I save lots of money by growing my own vegetables. But this isn't really true. In fact, if you added up all the hours I spend working in my garden and all the money I spend on things like seeds, gardening books, fertilizers, and plastic netting to keep the birds off the peas, each pound of peas I get out of my garden probably costs me about fifty bucks.

You may be asking yourself what in the world my expensive hobby of growing vegetables has to do with boys and puberty. The answer is, nothing at all. Except maybe for this one thing: each of the plants in my garden has its own way and time of growing. I have never been able to figure out why this is so. I can take two seeds from the same package that look exactly alike and plant them in the same row of my garden right next to each other. I will give them both the exact same amount of water, and they will both get the same amount of sunshine. Yet one seedling will come popping out of the ground and grow to a height of three or four inches before the other one has barely even broken through the top layer of soil. Boys, too, seem to have their own way and time of growing. One may start to go through puberty when he is only ten. Another might not start until he is fourteen.

The so-called "average" or "normal" or "regular" age at which boys start to go through puberty is around eleven or twelve. But very few boys are what we call average. The boys you see in Illustration 8 are both twelve years old. Both are completely healthy, normal, regular boys; however, one boy has already developed quite a bit. He has obviously started puberty. He has already gotten quite tall. He has grown a lot of pubic hair. His body has lots of muscles, and his penis and scrotum have grown quite a bit too. The other boy has barely even started to go through the body changes of puberty.

No one is sure why some boys start to go through puberty at a fairly young age and others do not start until they are older. It probably has something to do with a boy's family. If both your mother and father come from families in which people tend to start puberty at an early age, you probably will too. Or if both your parents come from familes in which people do not go through puberty until they are older, then you probably won't start to go through puberty until later too. This is not a hard and fast rule. A boy may be a later starter even if his parents were early starters. The opposite may also be true. But parents and children are

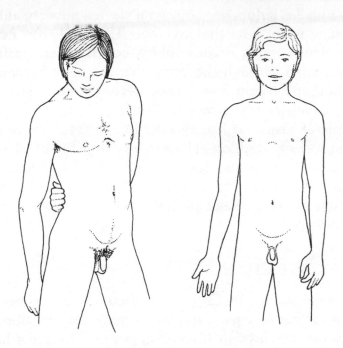

Illustration 8. Two twelve-year-olds. Both these boys are twelve. One has already developed quite a bit. The other hasn't begun to go through the body changes of puberty.

often alike in this way. You might want to ask your mom and dad how old they were when they started puberty.

Once a boy starts to go through the body changes of puberty, he may develop rather quickly or he may develop more slowly. I have noticed that the first seedlings to pop up in my garden always seem to be a step ahead of the other seedlings. They develop into fully grown, ripe plants before the others and are ready to be harvested first. A lot of people think that the same kind of thing holds true for boys going through puberty. They figure that the boys who start early will always be a step ahead of the other boys and will develop grown-up, adult bodies before the boys who started puberty at the average age or later than average. This isn't true, however. How young or how old a boy is when he first starts to go through the body changes of puberty has nothing to do with how fast he develops. Early starters may develop very grown-up looking bodies in just a couple of years, or it may take five years or more for them to fully develop. The same is true for boys who are late starters, and for boys who start at the more usual age of eleven or twelve. They may be quick, slow, or just about average in how fast they go through puberty.

THE FIRST CHANGES

As we explained in Chapter 1, there are a number of changes that take place in a boy's body during puberty. Boys can go through these changes in different order. For some boys, the first change that happens is that they begin to grow pubic hair. For most boys, though, the first change that takes place during puberty is that their sex organs begin to grow. This usually happens before they begin to develop pubic hairs, grow taller, or go through the other changes that take place during puberty. As puberty continues, the sex organs—the penis, scrotum, and testicles—continue to grow larger.

THE FIVE STAGES OF GENITAL DEVELOPMENT

Doctors have divided the growth and development of the genital, or sex, organs into the five stages shown in Illustration 9. You may be in one of these stages, or you may be in between one stage and another. See if you can find the stage you are closest to.

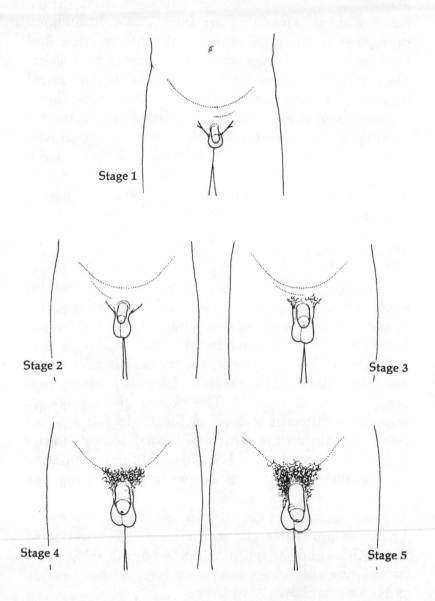

Illustration 9. The five stages of male genital development

Stage 1

Stage 1 starts when you are born and continues all through your childhood years. Your penis, scrotum, and testicles do not change very much during this stage. They may get a little bit larger in size, but all in all there is not much change in the way your genitals look.

Some boys have soft, light-colored, straight hair growing in their genital area during this stage. If you have this kind of hair, it will probably look pretty much like the hair you may have growing on your belly or legs or other parts of your body. But you won't have any dark- colored, curly pubic hair yet.

Stage 2

Stage 2 is the beginning of puberty. During this stage, the testicles get larger and the scrotal sac begins to hang lower. Of course, your testicles have been getting a bit larger all through childhood (Stage 1). But once puberty starts, they grow at a faster rate.

As the testicles get larger, the scrotal sac gets longer and hangs lower. The scrotum also gets looser, "baggier," and more wrinkly. The skin of the scrotal sac takes on a different texture, or "feel." In fair-skinned boys, the skin on the penis and scrotal sac gets rather reddish. Darker-skinned boys, too, will notice that the skin on their genitals gets deeper in color during this stage.

The penis doesn't get much larger during this stage. The most noticeable change in Stage 2 is the size of the testicles and the scrotum. Some boys develop pubic hair during this stage, but many boys do not develop pubic hair until Stage 3 or later.

As we explained, different boys begin puberty at different ages. Most boys start Stage 2 at about eleven or twelve, although some start when they are a year or so younger, and some when they are a year or so older than this.

For some boys, it is very clear when they have reached Stage 2 and started puberty. One day they look at their testicles and think, "Oh, wow, they've really gotten bigger." Other boys, especially those who have been watching their bodies closely, are not so sure. They may think, "It *seems* like they're getting bigger, but maybe I'm just imagining it."

Still other boys get to feeling kind of discouraged because puberty seems to be happening so slowly to them. They're eager to have mature, muscular bodies, and all that's happening is a little bit of growth in their testicles. If you start feeling down in the dumps because your body isn't changing as fast as you'd like, it helps to remember that all those changes you're waiting for *will* eventually happen.

If you're not certain if you've begun Stage 2, you might want to take a look at the orchidometer in Illustration 10. This is an actual, life-size drawing of an orchidometer, a tool doctors invented to study the different stages of puberty. It is a rather specialized tool, though, and not every doctor has one. It is a series of wooden or plastic egg-shaped ovals that are strung together on a cord in order of increasing size, from the smallest to the largest. If you were to hold the orchidometer in one hand and one of your testicles in the other hand, you would be able to see which of the ovals is closest in size to your testicle. Maybe you can get an idea of which you are closest to just by looking at the drawing and feeling one of your testicles.

The number written on each oval of the orchidometer shows the volume of that oval. *Volume* means "how

orchidometer (OR-ki-DOM-e-ter)

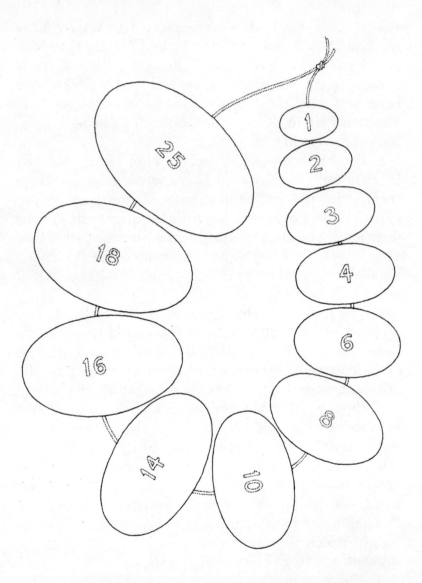

Illustration 10. Orchidometer, actual size

much something can hold," and it is a way of measuring size. The first oval on the orchidometer, the one marked 1, has a volume of one milliliter, which is about one-fifth of a teaspoon. The last oval, the one marked 25, has a volume of twenty-five milliliters, or about five teaspoons.

Fully grown men have testicles between sixteen and twenty-seven milliliters in volume. Boys who have not yet started puberty—that is, boys who are only in Stage 1—have testicles that are about the size of the 1, 2, or 3 ovals. If your testicle is the size of the 4 oval or larger, this means that you have reached Stage 2 and have officially begun puberty.

Stage 3
By the time a boy reaches Stage 3, his penis has begun to get bigger too. As you can tell from Illustration 9, the penis gets quite a bit larger than it was in Stage 1 or 2. It gets both longer and wider. The scrotum and testicles also grow during this stage, but the most noticeable change is in the size of the penis. The skin of the penis and scrotum also continues to deepen in color.

By the time a boy's penis has started to grow larger, his testicles are usually between seven and sixteen milliliters in volume (see the orchidometer in Illustration 10), although some boys in Stage 3 have testicles that are larger or smaller than this.

One testicle usually hangs lower than the other. In most grown men, it is the left testicle that hangs lower, but in some it is the right. If you have not noticed one testicle hanging lower than the other by the time you get to Stage 3, you will probably notice it during this stage.

The reason one testicle hangs lower than the other is to keep them from crushing each other when you walk.

If you have ever been hit in the testicles, you know that they are *very* sensitive. It can be really painful if your testicles get crushed together or if you get hit there. That is why boys often wear jockstraps or cup-shaped protectors in gym class or when they are playing sports (see Illustration 11). The jockstrap or cup holds the testicles snugly up against the body so that they are not hanging out and are protected from injury.

In grown men, both testicles are just about the same size, although sometimes one may be just a bit larger than the other. As you are developing, you may notice that one testicle is a good bit larger than the other. This is because one testicle may grow a bit faster. Often, the one that hangs lower is the largest. As the other grows, it may start to hang lower. So a boy who notices that his right testicle hangs lower in Stage 3 may find that his left testicle hangs lower in Stage 4. (If you are concerned about the difference in the size of your testicles or notice a sudden, dramatic change in size or in which

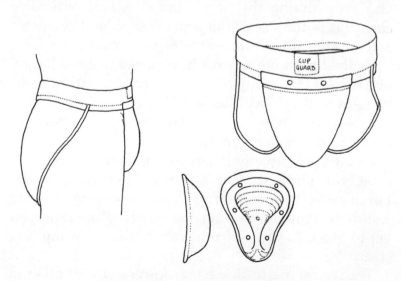

· **Illustration 11. Cup protector**

one is lowest, see the section on testicular self-examination, page 195.)

If a boy has not already started to develop pubic hair in Stage 2, he may notice the first curly hairs growing around the base of his penis during Stage 3. The first pubic hairs are not usually very dark in color or really curly. There aren't very many at first, and you may have to look very closely to see them. But as puberty continues, they will get darker in color and there will be more of them. They begin growing around the base of the penis, just where the penis joins the body. After a while, they start growing on the scrotum as well. They may also grow in the area around the anus.

Some of the boys and men we talked to were a bit worried when they started to grow pubic hair. Here is what some of them had to say:

> It looked like I was getting all these pimples on the skin around my cock.
>
> Jim, age 16

> There were little raised bumps, and I thought I had some kind of disease.
>
> Phil, age 24

> First I got these tiny, kind of whitish, raised spots. I was scared to say anything. I just waited. Then I noticed these fuzzy hairs growing out.
>
> Bill, age 17

When pubic hair starts to grow, there are often raised bumps on the surface of the skin that may look like pimples. These raised bumps are caused by the tiny pubic hairs trying to push through the skin. Soon, little hairs begin to poke through the surface of the bumps. If you don't know what is going on, it can be a bit scary. But it is a perfectly normal part of growing up, and it is not anything to worry about.

You may also notice that you have other little bumps or dots on the skin of the penis and scrotum, ones that do not grow little hairs. These are oil and perspiration (sweat) glands. They begin to develop during puberty and to make small amounts of oil and perspiration. You may notice that the skin in this area feels moister or smells a bit different. This is because your oil and perspiration glands are becoming active. Once again, this is a normal and natural part of growing up, another sign that you are becoming a man.

Just as it is impossible to say when a boy will reach Stage 2 and start puberty, so it is impossible to say when he will reach Stage 3. The usual age is about thirteen, although there are some who reach Stage 3 when they are younger than this, and some who reach it when they are older.

Stage 4

As you can see from Illustration 9 (page 47), by the time a boy reaches Stage 4, his penis has gotten quite a bit larger. It is both wider and longer, and the glans, or head, of the penis is more developed. The scrotum hangs lower and the testicles are also larger. The testicles are usually about 1½ inches long by the time a boy has reached this stage, and they are usually between twelve and twenty-four milliliters in volume (see Illustration 10)—although some boys' testicles will be slightly smaller or larger than this in Stage 4.

During this stage, the skin of the scrotal sac and penis continues to get deeper in color. The oil and sweat glands continue to develop too. The usual age at which boys reach Stage 4 is about fourteen, although again some boys will be younger than this and some will be older.

Most boys will have quite a bit of pubic hair by the

time they reach Stage 4. As a boy continues to develop, the pubic hair gets curlier, coarser, and darker in color. It usually grows in an upside-down triangle pattern on the lower part of his belly, around the base of the penis. In many boys, the pubic hair continues to grow up toward the belly button and out toward the thighs. As we mentioned before, it may also grow on the scrotum and around the anus.

Your pubic hair is often the same color as the hair on your head, but it may also be a lighter or darker color. When you become an old man, the pubic hair, like the hair on your head, is apt to turn gray.

Stage 5
This is the adult or fully grown stage. The testicles are usually about 1¾ inches long. They are generally between sixteen and twenty-seven milliliters in volume (see Illustration 10). The scrotal sac is also fully developed by the time a boy reaches this stage. And the skin of the scrotum and penis has gotten even deeper in color.

A grown man's penis is usually between 3¼ and 4¼ inches in length. When a man or boy has an erection, his penis gets temporarily larger. The largest erect penis ever recorded by a doctor was twelve inches long. The smallest was 4¾ inches. Ninety out of 100 men will have a penis that is between five and seven inches in length when it is erect, with the average length being about 6¼ inches. The smaller a penis is when it is soft, the more inches it tends to gain when it becomes erect. For example, a man with a penis that measures three inches when it is soft may add as many as 3¼ inches when his penis becomes hard. A man with a penis that measures 4¼ inches when soft might add only two inches during an erection. Thus, even though the lengths of their penises were different when they were soft, both men would have a 6¼-inch penis when they had erections. (We will talk more about penis size in Chapter 3.)

The penis may also get temporarily smaller from time to time. You may have noticed that your penis gets a little smaller if you jump into a cold bath or shower. Cold weather, being really tired out, or feeling nervous may also make your penis shrivel up a bit. Any of these things may also make your scrotal sac pull up closer to your body and seem temporarily smaller. In old age, the penis tends to become a bit smaller in size permanently.

The average age that boys reach Stage 5 is about sixteen, although as with Stages 1 through 4, there will be boys who enter Stage 5 when they are younger, and some when they are older.

The pubic hair is also fairly well developed by Stage 5. But pubic hair may continue to grow until the boy reaches the age of twenty.

Some boys have quite a bit of pubic hair; others have very little. How much you have will probably depend on your family. If the men in your family have lots of hair, you probably will too. If the men in your family are not especially hairy, chances are you will not be either. Again, this is not a hard and fast rule, but boys often take after their fathers in this way.

HOW LONG DOES IT TAKE TO GET THROUGH THESE STAGES?

There is no simple answer to this question because each boy is different. But doctors have studied boys going through puberty, so we can tell you about what happens to *most* boys.

As you may recall from the beginning of this chapter,

the earlier starters do not necessarily go through these stages any faster than boys who start puberty later or boys who start at the average age. Boys may take anywhere from a year to six years to go from Stage 2, the beginning of puberty, to Stage 5, the fully grown adult stage. The so-called average boy takes about four years. The table you see below shows how long boys take to go through each of the various stages of genital development. The first column shows how long the *average* boy takes to go through each stage. But, as we've said, not all boys are average. The second column shows the range of times it takes *most* boys to go through these stages.

THE LENGTH OF TIME BOYS SPEND IN STAGES 2, 3, AND 4

	The "Average" Boy	The Range of Times for 97 Out of 100 Boys
Stage 2	About 13 months	About 5 months to about 26 months
Stage 3	About 10 months	About 2 months to about 19 months
Stage 4	About 24 months	About 5 months to about 36 months

Let's say you are twelve years old and have just reached Stage 2. If you are a so-called typical or average boy, you will probably reach Stage 3 in about thirteen more months; that is, in one year and one month. However, you may be quick to develop and may find yourself in Stage 3 in only five months. Or you may be slower to develop and may not find yourself in Stage 3 until twenty-six months (two years and two months) have gone by. This table will not tell you exactly when the various changes that happen during puberty are going to happen to you, but it will give you some idea of what to expect.

FEELINGS ABOUT STARTING PUBERTY

Boys (and girls too) have all sorts of feelings about starting puberty. I've noticed that the kids in my youngest class (third and fourth graders), who haven't started puberty yet, are often excited about and looking forward to the changes that will take place in their bodies. But not everyone feels this way. As one third grader put it:

> Ugh! I don't want my penis to get all big and hairy and ugly looking!

By and large, though, the younger kids are really eager to grow up. They're curious about the changes that will take place and generally feel comfortable about asking questions in class. They don't use the Everything You Ever Wanted to Know question box as often as the older kids do. They just ask their questions right out loud.

The older kids who are about to start or have just started puberty are usually excited too. They often feel very proud when they notice their bodies starting to change. As one boy said:

> It's a "Hey, whoopee, I'm finally growing up!" kind of feeling.

But I've noticed that the older kids don't feel quite as comfortable about asking questions right out loud. As a group, they seem to feel more embarrassed about puberty than the younger kids. Even the kids who were in my class in third or fourth grade, and who were especially open and comfortable talking about the body changes of puberty, often seem more modest and rather shy about things by the time they're in sixth or seventh grade.

I think this difference I've noticed between the younger kids and the older ones is due, at least in part, to the fact that by the time you get to sixth or seventh grade, puberty is no longer some far-off thing that's going to happen someday. It's actually happening to *you*, and it's happening right now. It's much more personal, and this can make it harder to talk about.

I think, too, that once the changes have actually started to happen, most of us have some doubtful or uncertain feelings mixed in with our excited, proud feelings. Having mixed feelings about going through puberty is quite normal. Almost everyone has some doubts. One boy said it particularly well:

> I was taking a bath with my sister and she said, "What's that?" and I saw that I had some pubic hairs. I guess my penis and balls had been getting bigger all along. It wasn't till my sister saw the pubic hair that I really realized I was changing. I felt grown up and I was really jazzed about it. Then, two seconds later, I had this really scared feeling . . . "Oh, no, I'm not ready for this."

Many of the men and boys we interviewed remembered having these "I'm-not-ready" feelings. If you have these feelings, it helps to remember that it's quite normal to have them. In Chapter 8, we talk more about the kinds of feelings people have about going through puberty.

Some of the boys and men we talked to who started puberty late said that this had affected them. As one man explained:

> I didn't go through puberty until I was sixteen. It really bothered me when I was in situations where other boys

could see that I hadn't started yet. I was always embarrassed in gym class and I always tried to hide my body.

Jim, age 47

Another man told us:

I was a late starter, too. It seemed like all the other guys had really developed bodies and hair all over the place, and here I was still a skinny, little kid. Once it started, though, I really developed fast. My whole attitude was, "Thank God! At last it's happening to me." For a while there, I was thinking it would never happen and that maybe I was some kind of freak or maybe I was sick or there was something wrong. But, finally, I started to develop, too.

Glenn, age 42

Sometimes the boys and men who started earlier than the other guys had embarrassed feelings, too:

I developed at a very early age. I was really proud, but also embarrassed because I looked so different from the other kids. It's hard at that age to be different. You want to be just like the other guys and not stand out.

Pete, age 26

Even boys who started at the usual age sometimes felt embarrassed or uncertain about the changes taking place in their bodies, especially if they hadn't been told what to expect. Everyone we talked to, whether they felt proud and excited or uncertain and embarrassed (or a bit of both), agreed that it helps to have some idea of what to expect and to have someone to talk to about your feelings. Reading this book with someone might be a good way to start talking about these things.

AM I NORMAL?

As we're going through puberty, we may worry about whether everything is going according to plan. Sometimes puberty seems to be going very slowly. The changes in our bodies may be so slight as we move from stage to stage, especially in the early stages, that we wonder if we're really growing at all. We may ask ourselves, "Am I normal?" If you've started puberty, but your growth isn't as fast or dramatic as you'd like, hang in there. You *will* continue to grow and eventually you will have a fully mature adult body.

Boys who are late starters may also ask themselves, "Am I normal?" If they don't start puberty until two or three years after most of their friends have started, they often worry that maybe there's something wrong with them, that they have some kind of medical problem. But being a late starter doesn't usually mean there's anything physically wrong with you. It just means that your body is developing at a slower rate than most other boys' bodies.

Every once in a while, though, there are boys who are late starters not because they are simply slow to develop but because there is actually something physically wrong with them. Such boys need to see a doctor. Doctors have ways of treating these problems so that the boy will go through the normal body changes of puberty.

You may be wondering how you'd know if you were just a late starter or if you had a medical problem that needs a doctor's attention. We tell boys that if they've reached the age of fifteen and haven't started to go through any of the puberty changes described in this chapter, they should see a doctor. For example, a boy who was still in Stage 1 of genital development (see Illustration 9 on page 47) and who didn't have any pubic hair by age fifteen should see a doctor. Now, it doesn't necessarily mean that you have a medical problem if you haven't started to go through any of the body changes of puberty by the age of fifteen. There are some perfectly healthy boys who don't go through puberty until their late teens. But not starting by fifteen *may* mean you have a problem that needs medical attention, so it's a good idea to get it checked out.

By the way, if you have a feeling that something isn't right with the way your body is developing, you don't *have* to wait until you're fifteen to see a doctor. If you go to see a doctor before fifteen and it turns out that you do have a problem, you'll have caught the problem that much earlier. If you don't have a problem, you'll feel better knowing that you're just a late starter and that there's nothing wrong with you.

It's not just late starters who worry; boys who are early do too. But in most cases, being an early starter doesn't mean there's anything wrong with you. It just means that your body is developing a bit faster than other boys' bodies. However, just as being a late starter is occasionally a sign of a medical problem, so being an especially early starter can be a sign that something's wrong. If you begin puberty before the age of nine, it's a good idea to see a doctor to make sure that you don't have a problem.

KEEPING TRACK OF YOUR PROGRESS

Some of the boys in my classes get really interested in the stages of puberty. They study the five stages shown in Illustration 9 and compare their testicles to the orchidometer in Illustration 10. They pore over the

MY PUBERTY CHART

Date: _____
Height: _____ Weight: _____
Stage of Genital
Development: _____
Pubic Hair: _____
Facial Hair: _____
Other Changes: _____

_____

_____

_____

Date: _____
Height: _____ Weight: _____
Stage of Genital
Development: _____
Pubic Hair: _____
Facial Hair: _____
Other Changes: _____

_____

_____

_____

Date: _____
Height: _____ Weight: _____
Stage of Genital
Development: _____
Pubic Hair: _____
Facial Hair: _____
Other Changes: _____

_____

_____

_____

Date: _____
Height: _____ Weight: _____
Stage of Genital
Development: _____
Pubic Hair: _____
Facial Hair: _____
Other Changes: _____

_____

_____

_____

Date: _____
Height: _____ Weight: _____
Stage of Genital
Development: _____
Pubic Hair: _____
Facial Hair: _____
Other Changes: _____

_____

_____

_____

Date: _____
Height: _____ Weight: _____
Stage of Genital
Development: _____
Pubic Hair: _____
Facial Hair: _____
Other Changes: _____

_____

_____

_____

table on page 57 and try to figure out what stage they're at and when to expect other changes. Some of the boys in my class, however, couldn't care less. They figure that these changes are going to happen whether or not they pay attention to them, so why should they bother trying to follow it. You may be like the curious boys in my class, or you may be like those who are not as interested. If you *are* the type who likes to keep track of things, you might want to keep a record of your progress through puberty by using the chart on page 63. Before you fill out the chart, though, you might want to read the next few chapters, which talk about some of the other changes that happen to a boy's body during puberty.

How to Use the Puberty Chart

Start by filling in the first section of the chart. Write the date and record your height and weight. Then, turn back to Illustration 9 on page 47 and decide which stage of genital development you're closest to at the moment. Write the number of that stage on the appropriate line. On the Pubic Hair line, write "none" if you don't have any pubic hair yet. Or, if you have pubic hair already, write "a few hairs," "some dark, curly hairs," "lots of hair," or some other descriptive words. On the Facial Hair line, write "none" if you don't have any. If you've begun to develop a few dark hairs on the corner of your lip, your cheeks, or some other place, make a note on this line of the chart.

Some of the other puberty changes you might write about in the Other Changes section of the chart are:

body odor	breast swelling or tenderness
more erections	stronger sexual feelings
greater strength	more muscles
hairier arms and legs	oilier hair and skin
broader shoulders	voice changes
amount of perspiration	ejaculation
pimples	

Every three months or so, or every time you notice a big change, fill in a new section of the chart.

Keeping track of the changes that happen during puberty can give you more of a sense of being on top of things. It might be fun to do the chart with your mom or dad, with a friend, or with someone else close to you. Since fathers and sons are often alike in the way they go through puberty, you may want to keep this book and the charts you have filled in and pass them along to your own son if you have one someday.

CHAPTER 3

Changing Size and Shape

People often say that girls start puberty a year or two before boys, and I must admit that I used to think the same thing. I was really surprised to learn that the first puberty changes that take place in girls (the development of their sex organs, the growth of pubic hair, and the development of their breasts) happen at just about the same age that the first puberty changes in boys (the changes in the testicles, and the growth of pubic hair) begin to take place.

People get the idea that girls start puberty earlier than boys for two reasons. First of all, when a girl's breasts start to develop, we can see that this change is happening even though she is fully clothed. Most boys' testicles are starting to grow at the same time, but unless we see a boy naked, we are not aware of this change in his body in the way we are aware of a girl's breast development. Besides, the change in a boy's testicles is just not as dramatic as the changes that take place in a girl's body at the very beginning of puberty.

The second reason people think that girls go through puberty earlier than boys has to do with the "puberty growth spurt." During puberty, both boys and girls begin to grow taller at a faster rate, and a girl's growth spurt usually happens about two years before a boy's. This gives people the idea that girls start puberty before boys. But the growth spurt is just one of the changes that happen during puberty. The other puberty changes—things like the development of sex organs, of pubic hair, and, in girls, of the breasts—happen at about the same age in both boys and girls. Of course, some boys and girls are early starters and some are late starters, so everyone doesn't start at the same time. Still, the average boy and the average girl begin puberty at just about the same age.

THE GROWTH SPURT— WHEN AND HOW MUCH?

In girls, the growth spurt is sometimes the first change that happens during puberty. In boys, however, it rarely happens until the sex organs have begun to develop. Most boys start to notice the growth spurt between the ages of thirteen and fourteen, although some boys are somewhat younger or older when it starts.

Beginning at about the age of two, most children grow about two inches taller each year until they reach puberty. When the growth spurt begins, it may be very dramatic. Some boys add as many as five inches a year to their height during the growth spurt. Or the growth spurt may not be so sudden and noticeable. Some boys grow only about 2½ inches a year during the growth spurt. Most boys, though, grow about 3½ inches a year. The growth spurt may last for a few years. Then the rate of growth slows down again. This does not mean that a boy will stop growing altogether; most boys continue to grow taller until they get to about the age of twenty. But the period of extra-fast growth lasts only about three years.

HOW TALL WILL I BE?

A lot of boys want to know if there is any way that they can tell exactly how tall they will be when they are grown-up. Unfortunately, there isn't, but there are some clues that may help you make a rough guess. How tall you are usually has to do with your family. If both your parents are tall, chances are you will be too. If both your parents are short, you will probably be short. This is not a hard and fast rule, though—there are lots and lots of exceptions.

The tallest man who ever lived was eight feet, eleven inches tall, and the shortest was only 26½ inches. But these were unusual cases; 95 out of 100 Caucasian (white) and Negro (black) men will be between five feet, four inches and six feet, two inches tall. The average is five feet, nine inches tall.

By the way, don't make the mistake of thinking that boys who are on the short side before puberty will be shorter than the other men when they reach their adult heights. It is true that many boys who are short before puberty are short as adults, but this is not always the case. As one man said:

In eighth grade, I was the second-to-the-shortest kid in the class, but over the summer, I shot up. By the time I started ninth grade, I was just about the tallest boy in the class.

John, age 26

No one can say for sure which boys will end up being taller than average and which ones will end up being shorter than average—or, for that matter, which ones will end up being just about average. But we do know that by the age of ten, the average boy will have grown to 78 percent of his adult height and that by age fourteen, the average boy will have grown to 91.5 percent of his adult height. (*Percent* means "part of a hundred." A boy who reached his full height would have reached 100 percent of his adult height. A boy who had reached half his full height would have reached 50 percent of his adult height.)

CHANGING SHAPE

Illustration 12 shows an adult man and a baby boy. As you can see, we do quite a bit of growing between the time we're born and the time we reach our full adult size. For one thing, we get taller. As explained before, a lot of this growing taller happens during puberty. We also put on quite a bit of weight. At birth, the average boy baby weighs 7½ pounds. The average grown man weighs 162 pounds. Again, a lot of this weight gain happens during puberty.

If you compare the baby's body to the man's body, you'll see that some parts of the body grow more than others as we mature and grow into our adult bodies. If this weren't true, if all parts of our bodies grew the same amount as we matured, we'd simply grow into giant babies, and we'd look pretty strange. If you take a look at Illustration 13, you'll see what I mean.

Of course, we don't end up looking like giant babies. Different parts of our bodies grow more or less than other parts in proportion (in comparison to) other parts. For example, our heads don't grow as much as

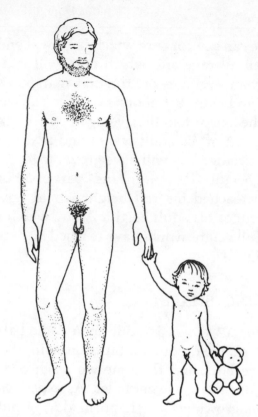

Illustration 12. Adult male and infant male

other parts of our body. During puberty, you may notice changes in the proportions or the size of certain
parts of your body in relation to other parts. For instance, the proportions of your face change. The lower
part gets longer, and this changes the general shape of
your face.

Your shoulders also get broader, and your hips seem
narrower in comparison to your broad shoulders. Your
shoulders become more muscular. In fact, the muscles
all over your body grow larger, especially in your
thighs, calves, and upper arms. With this increase in
the size of your muscles comes an increase in body

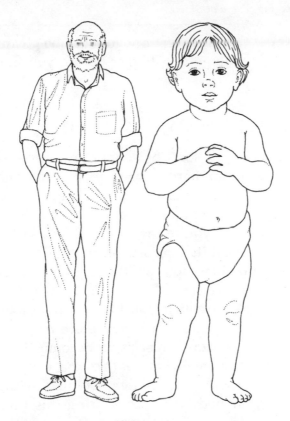

Illustration 13. Adult male and giant baby

strength. Your whole body begins to look less like a boy's body and more like a man's. Your arms and legs tend to grow faster than your backbone during your growth spurt. So you may notice that your arms and legs are longer in proportion to the trunk of your body than they were during childhood or than they are in adulthood. The bones in your feet also grow faster than your other bones, and so your feet usually reach their adult size before you reach your full height. Some boys whose feet are already quite large but who are still going through the growth spurt think that their feet are going to continue to grow as they get taller.

They worry that their feet are going to be gigantic. But your feet do stop getting bigger before you finish getting taller.

LIKING YOUR BODY

Bodies come in all sorts of shapes and sizes—short or tall, thin or plump, narrow or wide, muscular or not so muscular. To some extent, you can change the shape of your body by diet and exercise. If you're thin, you can put on weight. If you're fat, you can diet so that your body loses some if its fat tissue. If you'd like your body to be more muscular, you can lift weights or work out in a gym once you've started puberty. Doing slow, repetitious exercises, in which you lift weights or use your muscles to push against a heavy piece of gym equipment, will cause your muscles to become thicker and shorter and to bulge out more. (You have to wait until you've started puberty, though, because without the hormones your body produces during this time—we'll talk more about these in Chapter 4—your muscles won't respond to the exercise.) But remember that you do have a basic body shape that can't be changed no matter how much or how little you eat or what type of exercise you do.

If you aren't satisfied with your body and are under- or overweight, perhaps you need to see a doctor and get on a diet and exercise plan to help you gain or lose weight. If you are not sure whether you're under- or overweight, your doctor can help you decide if your weight is within the normal ranges for age, height, and body build. If you fall within the normal ranges and still aren't satisfied with the way your body looks, maybe you need to think about where you've gotten these ideas about how your body *should* look, ideas that are making you feel dissatisfied with the way you *do* look.

It would be nice if we could all just look at our bodies without having to compare them to someone else's and say, "Hey, I like the way I look." But we live in a society where there's a lot of competition among people, companies, and even countries. We're always comparing and competing to see who's best. So who decides what's best?

Most of us get our ideas about what's the "best" or "most attractive" kind of male body from the pictures we see in magazines, on billboards, and in television and the movies. Right now in our country, these pictures often show tall men with big, bulging muscles, handsome, regular features, no pimples, slim waists, small rear ends, and hairy chests. As you may have noticed, not too many men actually look like this.

When we are constantly bombarded with pictures of these tall, muscular, handsome men, we can get the feeling that there's something about our bodies that is somehow not right. If we don't look like them, we may be unhappy with the way we look. After all, if these are the men who are always the heros in the movies, always getting the girls or winding up being successful, what message does that send to those of us who aren't tall, muscular, or good-looking in that particular way? With all these images of perfect "hunks," it's easy to get to thinking that their bodies actually *are* better or more attractive. If you feel this way sometimes, it helps to remember that these bodies seem more desirable only because they are in fashion in our particular culture at this particular time. Being in fashion doesn't make a miniskirt "better" than a knee-length skirt, and being in fashion doesn't make one body type better than another.

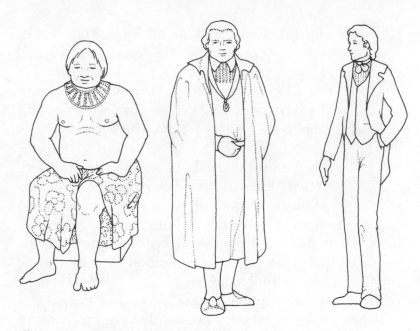

Illustration 14. Fashions in appearance. From the left are a Polynesian king, a seventeenth-century German burghermeister, and a nineteenth-century Englishman.

It helps, too, to remember that fashions change and that they vary from culture to culture. Illustration 14 shows bodies that have been in fashion in other times and other cultures. The first drawing is a Polynesian king. Most people in our society would find him grossly overweight, yet in his culture he's considered a fine figure of a man. His huge belly is taken as a sign of his masculinity. The seventeenth-century German burghermeister in the second picture would also be considered a bit chunky by our standards, yet in his own day and age his bulk was considered attractive, a sign of his success and prosperity. The third fellow is an Englishman from the nineteenth century. His thin, narrow body and lack of muscles make him look rather fragile in comparison to the hunk kind of body now in fashion in our country. Yet back then, in England, he was the type of guy who had women swooning over him. In fact, back then, one of our modern-day hunks might have been considered a real barbarian and not at all attractive.

It also helps to remember that not everyone agrees with or goes along with the fashions of the day. For instance, there are plenty of women who find men with huge muscles popping out all over grossly unattractive. Many women prefer thin men. And for most people, it's not what kind of body you have but what kind of person you are that really counts.

Learning to appreciate yourself and to like your own body, regardless of whether or not it matches up to what's in fashion, is a big step in growing up. If you find your own body attractive, other people will too.

Of course, it isn't always easy to learn to like your own body. Even though most of the boys we talked to were pleased about the fact that their bodies were changing and becoming adult, they sometimes wished that they were taller or wider across the chest, or more muscular, or more something else. We asked the men we interviewed, "Have you ever wished your body were different in some way, and if so, how?", or "What's the one thing you would most like to change about your body?" We got many different answers, but two topics came up more than the others, so we'd like to talk a bit about them.

Height
One thing that men mentioned over and over again was their height. Except for those who were very tall, almost all of the men we interviewed said they wished they

were a bit taller. Even if they were average height (five feet, nine inches) or a couple of inches taller than average, they often said they "wouldn't mind" being a bit taller. The men who were shorter than average almost always said they wished they were taller. As one man put it:

I'm only five feet, six inches, and being short has always bugged me. People make cracks, call you "shrimp" or "shortie." I'm really coordinated and good at sports. Being short made it difficult to get on the team in high school. I guess I compensated by getting into weight lifting and concentrating on wrestling. In a way, though, now that I'm older, it turns out that being short was kind of an advantage because it made really concentrating on working out and developing a strong, muscular body a habit that's stayed with me. I still work out and I'm in great physical shape, whereas a lot of guys my age, the ones who were tall in high school and all, are overweight and flabby and out of shape. I'm healthier than a lot of guys, and maybe if I'd been taller I wouldn't have gotten so into working out and taking care of my body. Still, to tell the truth, I still wish I were taller.

Harold, age 34

Another man had this to say:

No doubt about it, being tall is an advantage. People look up to you. I think being short is a disadvantage, in sports, with girls . . . and in other ways. Short guys have a lot of problems to contend with that just aren't there for tall guys.

Hank, age 20

Not all short men are bothered by their lack of height:

I've always been short, even as a kid, so I've had a whole lifetime to adjust, and it's really not a problem for me like it is for some guys. I know lots of short guys who are always kind of cocky, on the defensive, who talk loud or always act the clown or are kind of brash or pushy. They're sort of making up for the fact that they're short, acting big so that people will notice them, like they might get missed or passed over because they're short. But I don't really feel that need. I'm short and I'm a pretty quiet guy, but I still feel that people take note of me because I'm comfortable with myself the way I am. I think people notice or feel that kind of satisfaction when you're at peace with yourself and accept yourself the way you are.

Rick, age 39

And tall men aren't always happy about their height:

I'm six foot seven, and I'm always looking down on other people. People are always saying dumb things like, "How is the weather up there?" I was this tall when I was fourteen, and I always felt like a freak. I kind of slouched and hunched over, trying not to look so tall. My mother was always yelling at me to stand up straight. I still have terrible posture. I'm in my forties now, so it's not so bad anymore. There are little inconveniences, like bumping your head and trying to scrunch into cars, but it's not like when I was a teenager. It really bothered me then. Being different was difficult.

Frank, age 43

But being short can pose problems, as Rick explains:

There's a sort of unwritten rule that the guy has to be taller than the girl. All the girls were always taller than me, so I realized early on that I wasn't going to pay attention to that rule because if I only asked out girls who were shorter than me . . . well, I wouldn't have gone out on too many dates. So I just ignored that rule and asked out whomever I wanted. I got turned down sometimes, just on account of my height. There were girls, and later women, who even though they'd go out with me were bothered by my being short. They'd wear flat-heeled shoes instead of the high heels they probably would have worn. But once I got involved with someone, you know, seriously, we'd kid around and it was never a real problem. It's true that a lot of people follow this rule about the guy having to be taller, and it does affect you. Maybe it's a little harder to get a date, to find a girl who isn't uptight about it. My wife, by the way, is five inches taller than me and wears high heels, and it doesn't bother her that there's a difference in our height. It is breaking that unwritten law, though, and people do look at us. I figure that's their problem.

Rick, age 39

Rick has a healthy attitude about himself and doesn't seem to worry about what other people think. But there's no getting around the fact that our society attaches a lot of importance to a man's height. In fact, many people are prejudiced against short men. You're probably familiar with racial prejudice. People who have racial prejudices make judgments about or discriminate against people whose skin is a different color from theirs. They prejudge (*prejudice* means "to prejudge") people of other races and make assumptions about what they are like before they even meet or get to know anything about them as individuals. Prejudice against short men isn't as obvious or as talked about as racial prejudice, but it does exist and can cause problems. For example, studies have shown that if two equally qualified men apply for a job and one is tall and the other short, the tall man is more likely to get the job, simply because he's tall.

In other studies, researchers have given people pictures of a tall man and a short man and asked them to write descriptions of what they think these men are like based on the pictures. The researchers found that people tend to describe the tall man in more positive terms, using words like "brave," "sincere," "handsome," "successful," and so on. They tend to describe the short man in less positive or even negative terms: "not so successful," "insecure," "dishonest," and so forth.

Given the kinds of prejudices some (not all, but some) people have, it's not surprising that short men often wish they were taller. The truth of the matter is that your height doesn't have anything to do with your worth as a person, and it doesn't have anything to do with how successful you may become. Think of the many shorter-than-average men who have become famous stars, men like actors Dustin Hoffman and Dudley Moore, and baseball greats Phil Rizzuto and Joe Morgan, among many others. Of course, knowing this fact intellectually is a lot easier than really believing it with your heart and feeling okay about yourself if you're short. It helps to remember what Rick said about people responding to a person who has the inner satisfaction and confidence that comes from accepting himself the way he is. It's true. If you learn to accept yourself, to take pride in your unique self, then other people will too.

Penis Size

The other thing that often came up when we asked men how they felt about their bodies was the issue of penis size. Perhaps you've heard people make jokes about this subject. Or maybe you have been in the showers in the gym locker room and heard boys teasing other boys about the size of their penis. Maybe you have done this kind of teasing yourself, or you have been teased in this way.

If any of these things have happened to you, you're not alone. However, you may never have heard these sorts of jokes or teasing, or wished your penis were larger. If this is the case, you may be wondering what all the fuss is about.

People often make a big deal out of penis size because they believe the many myths that they hear about it. Myths are stories that people believe are true, but, as we shall see, many myths are completely false. Here are some of the myths that people tell about penis size, along with the real facts.

Myth: Tall men with big, husky builds and lots of muscles have bigger penises than short or skinny men.

Fact: The size of your penis doesn't have anything to do with how tall you are, how muscular you are, how much you weigh, or how your body is built. A short skinny man may have a big penis or a small one. A tall husky football player may have a big one or a small one.

Myth: Men with big thumbs have big penises. This myth has many variations: men with big noses, big ears, big feet . . . men with big whatevers.

Fact: The size of your penis has nothing to do with the size of any other part of your body. No one can tell what size your penis is by looking at the size of your thumb, your nose, your feet, your ears, or any other part of your body.

Myth: Men who come from a certain racial or ethnic background have bigger penises. Sometimes this myth specifies a certain race or ethnic group. For example, you may have heard that black men or Italian men have bigger penises.

Fact: There is no scientific evidence to show that men belonging to any one racial or ethnic group have larger penises than men from other races or ethnic groups.

Myth: A man whose penis is shorter than usual when soft has a shorter-than-average penis when erect.

Fact: The size of your penis when it is soft does not really have much to do with the size it is when it is erect. As we explained in Chapter 2, most grown men's penises are about 3¼ to 4¼ inches long when they are soft. Those that are on the short size when they are soft, say 3¼ inches or so, may add about three inches when they are erect. Men whose penises are on the long side, say 4¼ inches, may get only about two inches more during an erection. However, almost everyone, regardless of the size of their penis when soft, adds at least two inches when they are having an erection. So a man whose penis is unusually large when it is soft, say seven inches, might have a nine-inch penis when it is hard. Most men's penises are about 6¼ inches long when they are having an erection, regardless of how long they are when they are soft.

Myth: Men with big penises are more masculine, or "manly," or macho than men with smaller penises. This myth has many variations, depending on what people consider manly or masculine. You may have heard that men who have large penises are better at sports, or braver, or stronger.

Fact: The size of your penis does not have anything to do with how brave or strong or masculine or manly you are.

Myth: Men with big penises make more sperm in their bodies and can get a woman pregnant more easily than men with smaller penises.

Fact: The size of your penis or, for that matter, your testicles has nothing to do with how many sperm your testicles make. If a man with a big penis has sexual intercourse with a woman, she is not any more or less likely to get pregnant than if she had had sex with a man with a small penis.

Myth: If your penis is small, it won't "fit" into a woman's vagina when you are having sexual intercourse. You may also have heard the opposite of this myth: that if a man's penis is too big, it won't fit into the woman's vagina.

Fact: There are certain very rare medical conditions that can cause a man's penis to be abnormally small or abnormally large. But other than these one-in-a-million cases, penises are never too large or too small for a man to have intercourse with a woman. A woman's vagina is only about three inches long, but it is very expandable. If you recall from Chapter 1, a woman's vagina can expand enough to allow a baby to pass through it when she is giving birth. Babies weigh anywhere from about five to ten pounds when they are born, so they are considerably larger than any man's penis. It is just not true that a man's penis can be too large.

A woman's vagina is like a balloon with no air in it. The sides rest up against each other, just as the sides of a collapsed balloon do. So even if a man had a very small penis, it would still fit snugly inside a woman's vagina.

Myth: Men with big penises are more sexually powerful. This myth also has many variations: men with big penises have a stronger sexual drive, have a larger sexual appetite, have more erections, or have erections that last longer.

Fact: The size of your penis does not have anything to do with any of these things. Different men have different sexual drives, and some have erections more often than others, but these differences have nothing to do with their penis size.

Myth: Women enjoy sex more if the man has a big penis.

Fact: Penis size has very little to do with how much a woman enjoys sexual intercourse. Women's pleasure in intercourse comes mostly from the stimulation they get in the area around the clitoris and the vaginal opening, rather than inside the vagina. So the size of the penis is of little importance.

With all these myths going around, it's not surprising that men often worry about whether their penis is "big enough" or wish that it were larger. If you've worried about this, it helps to remember that all of these myths are simply that—myths. *They just aren't true.* The size of your penis doesn't have anything to do with how much of a man you are or what kind of a person you are.

We hope that the information we've given you so far will help you feel easier about the changes taking place in your body. We hope it will help you learn to accept and like your body, regardless of whether you're tall or short, have a big penis or a small one, are muscular or aren't so muscular. Remember, it's the person inside the body, not the body itself, that's important. If you learn to feel good about your body, other people will too.

CHAPTER 4

Body Hair, Whiskers, Beards, Mustaches, Perspiration, Pimples, and Other Puberty Changes

---

If the increase in the size of your penis and testicles and the growth spurt were the only things that happened during puberty, Dane and I could have ended this book right here. But, as you may have guessed, there are also other changes that go on in your body during puberty. In this chapter and the next, we will be talking about some of these other changes.

THE ROLE OF HORMONES

You may be wondering what causes all these changes. The fact of the matter is that no one knows for sure, but we do know that it has something to do with *hormones*. Hormones are substances that are made by parts of our bodies called glands. The hormones made in our various glands travel to other parts of our bodies and tell those parts how to develop and grow, or how to work and behave properly.

Our bodies have a number of different glands making dozens of different hormones, most of which have long, tongue-twisting names that you can hardly pronounce, let alone spell. You could go crazy trying to remember the names of all these glands and hormones. But we don't want you to go crazy, so we're only going to talk about the glands and hormones that have the most to do with puberty.

Puberty starts in your brain. A few years before your sex organs start to grow larger or you start to go through your growth spurt, glands in your brain start making larger and larger amounts of certain hormones. One of these glands in your brain is called the *pituitary gland*. The pituitary makes a hormone that gets into your bloodstream and travels to your testicles. As you get older, your pituitary sends more and more of its hormones to your testicles. Your testicles are also glands. The hormones from your brain cause your testicles to make hormones of their own. The most important hormone your testicles make is *testosterone*.

As you begin to go through puberty, your testicles (in response to greater amounts of brain hormones) make increasing amounts of testosterone. The testosterone travels to other parts of your body and tells those parts how to grow and develop. For instance, it is testosterone that causes your penis, testicles, and scrotum to

hormones (HOR-moans)
pituitary (pih-TOO-eh-tearee)
testosterone (tes-tos-TUR-own)

grow larger. Testosterone is also responsible for the growth of those curly, crisp pubic hairs. In fact, testosterone plays a role in almost all of the changes we will be talking about in this chapter and the next.

BODY HAIR

In addition to those curly pubic hairs, testosterone also causes hair to grow on other parts of your body. As you're going through puberty, you may notice that you have more hair on your arms, your thighs, and your lower legs. This hair probably won't be as curly as your pubic hair. But there will usually be more hair in these areas of your body than there was during childhood. Hair may also start to grow on your chest. Some boys grow hair on their shoulders and/or their backs. Some grow hair on the backs of their hands. Some boys become really hairy; others have very little body hair.

People often think that the amount of body hair a man has is related to how much testosterone his testicles make. This isn't true. Testosterone causes your body hair to *start* to grow, but how much or how little a man has doesn't have anything to do with how much testosterone his body makes. The amount of body hair you'll have is determined by two things: your racial or ethnic group and your family. As a group, Caucasian (white) men generally have more body hair than Oriental or Negro (black) men. Within any of these groups, the amount of hair a man has usually depends on his family. Boys who come from families in which the men tend to have lots of hair usually wind up having a lot of body hair. Boys who come from families in which the men have little or no hair on their chests, arms, legs, hands, and so forth usually have very little hair. Once again, this isn't a hard and fast rule, but hairiness (or lack of hair) does tend to, as they say, "run in families."

Just as there are a lot of myths about penis size, so there are a lot of myths about body hair. Some people believe that men who have a lot of body hair are more manly or masculine than men who don't have so much. This is nonsense. Body hair (or lack of body hair) doesn't have anything to do with how much of a man you are. Some people (both men *and* women) find lots of body hair attractive. For them, body hair is especially sexy. Others feel that smoother, more hairless bodies are more attractive. But for most people, it doesn't matter that much one way or the other. So if you've worried about the amount of body hair you have, you probably shouldn't bother. For one thing, worrying won't make any difference. Besides, anyone who is going to decide whether or not they like you on the basis of how much body hair you have probably isn't worth knowing anyhow.

FACIAL HAIR

As a boy goes through puberty, he also starts to grow hair on his face. His mustache, sideburns, whiskers, and beard begin to develop. The first of this facial hair doesn't usually appear until a boy's sex organs are fairly well-developed, usually during Stage 4 of genital development (see Illustration 9 on page 47). The average boy will develop his first facial hair between the ages of fourteen and sixteen. A few boys, though, will notice this hair before they're thirteen, and some don't get any until they're nineteen or twenty.

Usually, the first facial hairs will appear at the outer corners of your upper lip. In the beginning, they may be only slightly dark in color and there will only be a few of them. As you get older, they will get deeper in color and there will be more of them. Your mustache will gradually fill out, growing from the outer corners toward the middle of your lips. At about the same time that your mustache is growing in, hairs usually being to grow on the upper part of your cheeks and just below the center of your lower lip. Your sideburns may also grow at this time.

As you continue to mature, your facial hair will get thicker and darker in color. Your beard and mustache may be the same color as the hair on your head, or they may be a different color. You may find that by age eighteen, your beard and mustache are as full and thick as they're ever going to be. However, many men don't develop their full facial hair until ten years after they have completed puberty and reached their full adult height. Many a man finds that he can grow a thick beard or a bushy mustache and sideburns at age thirty, even though he hardly had any facial hair when he was in his teens or early twenties.

Shaving

Some grown men shave off their facial hair every day or even twice a day (if they have thick, fast-growing hair). Others will let their mustaches, sideburns, and/ or beards grow and only trim them every once in a while to keep them neat. Still others just let their facial hair grow and only rarely, if ever, shave or trim it. It is a personal thing, a matter of individual taste.

Many of the men we talked to shaved when their facial hair first started to grow, even if later in life they decided not to shave. One mustached man said:

I don't shave it now. When I was a teenager I did, though —because it was just these few scrawny hairs. It looked pretty pathetic; kind of scraggly. It didn't look like a real mustache.

Phil, age 30

Another man said:

I don't shave anymore, just too lazy to shave every day. When I got that first peach fuzz, I shaved every day, religiously. It was kind of a macho thing. Also, I don't know if it's true or not, but I heard the more you shave, the faster your mustache and beard would grow in.

Ted, age 36

(By the way, Ted is probably right. Shaved hairs tend to grow back darker and thicker.)

A lot of the boys we talked to felt excited about shaving and looked upon shaving as a sign of growing up. Many boys wished they had as much facial hair as some of their friends had. One man told a funny story about this:

I ran around with my cousin, Albert, and his gang, who were all in their mid-twenties. I was, say, nineteen. Albert had a car, a Model-T, which was something—having a car that is—in those days. So it was really exciting for me to run around with these older guys. I wanted to look as old as them, so I'd get my mother's eyebrow pencil and color my mustache in, you know, to make me look more mature.

So we go to a dance, and afterward I'm smooching with this gal in the back seat of Albert's car, and my mustache smears off all over her face. Jeez, talk about embarrassing. I thought I'd never live it down!

Charlie, age 67

Getting their first razor was also a big event for some boys. Some bought these razors themselves; others got theirs as gifts. Some used their dad's razor at first:

When I first started shaving, I didn't say anything to anyone. I didn't want to buy one [a razor] and just leave it there in the bathroom 'cause I knew my family would just tease me to death about it. I really didn't have that much to shave. So I just used my dad's razor.

My sisters were starting to shave their legs, and they were using dad's razor, too. He'd get hopping mad 'cause he'd go to shave his face and the blade would be dull and nicked 'cause my sisters and I used it all the time. He'd cut his face all up and then he'd start hollerin', "Who's been using my razor?" My sisters and I would say, "Not me, not me!" Finally he went out and bought us all razors and told us, "You kids use my razor again and I'll kill you."

Sam, age 35

If you do start to shave, make sure that the blades of your razor are smooth and free of nicks, or you're apt to cut yourself. A dull blade can pull at your skin and irritate it, so make sure you've got a sharp one. But go easy—you can cut yourself with a sharp blade. Using soap or shaving cream will ease the pull or drag of the razor on your skin. There are also electric razors. You're a lot less likely to cut yourself with an electric razor, but some men don't like them. You might talk to your dad or another adult male to find out what he recommends for shaving.

UNDERARM HAIR AND PERSPIRATION

At about the same time that you start growing facial hair, you'll probably notice hair growing under your armpits. Occasionally, there's a boy who develops underarm hair before he begins to grow a mustache or even before he develops pubic hair. But for most boys, facial hair and underarm hair appear at about the same time.

Once you begin to grow underarm hair, or even before, you may notice that your underarms perspire (sweat) more, and that your perspiration has a different odor from when you were younger. You may also notice that other areas of your body, such as your genitals and your feet, have a different odor. Or you may notice that your hands tend to perspire and get rather clammy from time to time.

These changes happen because the testosterone from your testicles affects the perspiration glands located in these areas of your body. It is all a natural, healthy part of growing up, but some teenagers worry about the smells and the increase in perspiration. Actually, it's not too surprising that some teenagers are concerned. Advertising agencies spend millions of dollars each year on TV commercials designed to make us worry about our body odors and whether or not we're "dry" enough. But if you're eating properly and are healthy, your body odor probably isn't offensive. Bathing or showering regularly and wearing freshly laundered clothes should keep you smelling clean and fresh. If you perspire quite a bit and this bothers you, you may find that wearing 100 percent cotton undershirts and shorts will help. Cotton is more absorbent than synthetic (man-made) materials. Wearing outer shirts and pants made of cotton or wool or other natural fibers may also help.

We all tend to perspire more when we're nervous. During puberty, this tendency may be even more noticeable. Lots of teenagers get clammy hands or break out in a sweat when they get uptight. This is perfectly normal and usually lessens after you reach your twenties. If you have this problem, it helps to remember that it is normal. Sometimes just admitting to yourself, "Yup, I'm feeling really nervous (or embarrassed or uptight) right now," will help you relax and perspire less.

Deodorants and Antiperspirants

If you are bothered by the odor or amount of your perspiration, you may want to use a deodorant and/or an antiperspirant. There are a number of these products on the market. They come in aerosol cans, non-aerosol sprays, sticks, creams, roll-ons—you name it. Some are "unscented," and some have a scent added to cover up the smell of the product. Some are advertised as being "a man's deodorant," but there generally isn't much difference between a so-called man's deodorant and a woman's deodorant.

Deodorants are aimed at covering up your body odor with the supposedly more pleasant odor of the deodorant. Antiperspirants also have a substance to dry up perspiration. The most effective antiperspirants have a substance called aluminum chlorohydrate. Some people think that the aluminum can soak through your skin and get into your bloodstream, and that this may be harmful. Other people disagree. You'll have to decide for yourself whether you want to use this kind of product.

Whatever you decide, be sure to read the label. Some products work best when you use them at bedtime rather than first thing in the morning. You may find that it is better not to put the deodorant or antiperspirant on just after you jump out of a hot shower. If you perspire after the shower, the deodorant/antiperspirant may just wash away. It might be better to let your body cool down a bit first.

With the way we've been going on about deodorants and perspiration here, you may be thinking, "Oh, wow, I'd better run right out and get some." Please remember, though, that body smells are natural and normal, and unless your odor or the amount of perspiration bothers you, it's not really necessary to use anything.

SKIN CHANGES

At the same time that your perspiration glands are becoming more active, your body's oil glands are also working harder. As we explained in Chapter 2, more oil will be produced by the glands in your genital area, and this may make the skin of your penis and scrotum feel somewhat moist. The oil glands in your scalp may also start producing more. You may find that your hair gets more oily or greasy and that you have to shampoo it more often.

Pimples, Acne, and Other Skin Disturbances

The oil glands in your skin are also affected by the hormones your body starts making during puberty. Your skin becomes more oily, and for many boys and girls, this leads to skin problems like pimples. Some boys and girls have only mild problems with their skin; others have more severe problems; still others don't have problems at all. But eight out of every ten teenagers have at least mild skin problems, and boys seem to be even more susceptible than girls.

Pimples and other skin disturbances happen because the hormones, such as testosterone, that your body begins making during puberty cause your oil glands to make excess amounts of a substance called *sebum*. You have oil glands all over your skin. They are especially numerous on your face, neck, shoulders, upper chest, and back. Illustration 15 shows an oil gland. Sebum is made in the lower part of the gland and travels through the duct to the *pore*, the opening on the surface of your skin.

sebum (SEE-bum)

If you're producing a great deal of sebum, the pore may become clogged, and a blackhead may form. A lot of people think that blackheads are little particles of dirt trapped in the pores. This isn't true. Blackheads are black not from dirt but because the sebum and other substances produced by the glands sometimes turn black when they come in contact with the oxygen in the air.

Some boys and girls get whiteheads, which are also the result of sebum. The sebum gets trapped just below the surface of the skin and forms the small, raised whitish bumps we call whiteheads.

If blackheads are not removed, the sebum may continue to fill the duct. This may cause pressure, irritation, and inflammation. Germs can get in the duct and cause an infection. Whiteheads are also inflamed and infected. Pimples—red bumps that may be filled with whitish pus and that many teenagers call "zits"—may develop. If you have a serious case of pimples, you may have a

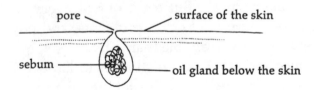

We have tiny oil glands just below the surface of our skin. These oil glands produce an oily substance called sebum.

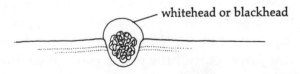

During puberty, our oil glands begin producing more sebum. If the pore, or opening, to the gland becomes blocked, a pimple may form.

Illustration 15. Oil gland

problem called *acne*. Acne can be very troublesome and may cause pitting or scarring of the skin.

Pimples and acne are often more of a problem for those who naturally tend to have more oily skin. The oiliness of your skin type, plus the increased oil you produce during puberty, combine to make you a candidate for these kinds of skin problems. If you have oily skin and acne during your teen years, you may find yourself wishing you had drier, less acne-prone skin. But when you're older, you may be glad to have oily skin, because this type of skin doesn't wrinkle as easily as dry skin does.

Acne also tends to "run in families," so if your parents or older brothers and sisters had acne, you may be more likely to develop it. Many doctors believe that eating certain foods—chocolate, salty foods like nuts and chips, and greasy foods—make a person more susceptible to acne. However, some doctors disagree. In one study, the amount of chocolate eaten didn't seem to have anything to do with acne. Still, if you find that certain foods give you pimples, it's best to avoid those foods.

Stress may also be a factor in acne. A lot of teens find that they "break out"—that is, get a lot of pimples —just before an important event—a dance, a big date, a game—that they're particularly nervous or excited about.

Although sunlight may have a beneficial effect on acne and help to "dry out" your skin, it may also aggravate the problem. If you live in a hot dry climate like that found in California, the sunshine may be helpful. However, hot humid (moist) climates, such as those of Hawaii or Florida, may make your acne even worse.

acne (AK-nee)

Some teens sit under a sunlamp to help dry out their acne and/or to get a tan. This isn't always a good idea. For one thing, sitting under a sunlamp can cause a severe sunburn, even if you only sit there for a minute more than the recommended time. While you're under the lamp, it may not seem like much is happening, so it's tempting to stay longer. All too often, this results in red, sunburned skin the next day. If you use a sunlamp, *follow the instructions carefully*. Another problem with sunlamps, or for that matter, with prolonged sunbathing, is that it can cause your skin to age before its time. People who have spent a lot of time in the sun or under sunlamps may be wrinkly and look like they're fifty or sixty by the time they're thirty. Overexposure to sunlight also increases your chances of getting skin cancer later in life. So be sure to go easy on the sun and tanning treatments.

Acne is most common between the ages of fourteen and seventeen, although it also happens to older and younger boys and girls. In boys, it tends to be worse during Stages 3 and 4 of genital development.

Some teens are troubled by acne for only a year or two. Then their oil glands adjust themselves to the hormones, their skin becomes less oily, and their acne and pimples clear up. Others have these problems throughout their teenage years. For a few boys and girls, acne continues to be a problem even after their teens.

The kids in my class generally want to know if there is anything they can do to prevent pimples or to cure acne. I explain that although there aren't any foolproof ways to prevent pimples, or any 100 percent effective cures for acne, there are some things that help many teens. Frequent shampoos will keep greasy, oily hair from adding to the oil on your skin. Washing the especially oily areas—your face, neck, shoulders, back, and upper chest—at least once a day may also help prevent pimples. Washing removes the oil from the surface of the skin and helps keep your pores open. Wash with hot water, which helps open your pores, and rinse with cold water to close the pores up again. Wiping with a pad soaked in isopropyl alcohol after you wash will remove any leftover oil and dirt. You can buy isopropyl alcohol for under fifty cents a bottle in a drugstore, and use cotton balls or pads. You can also buy special presoaked pads, but they're usually rather expensive. Go easy with the alcohol, though. It can remove too much oil and leave your skin too dry.

If you have especially oily skin, you may want to wash two or three times a day with ordinary soap. If you tend to get pimples, one of the antibacterial soaps sold in drugstores and pharmacies may help. (Ask the druggist to recommend one.) If you have pimples on your back, shower once or twice a day using an antibacterial soap and a back brush to scrub.

If you have blackheads, an abrasive soap or cleanser may help. (Again, ask your druggist to recommend one.) The abrasive in the soap often removes the blackheads and opens your pores. Be careful, though, because these soaps can irritate your skin. Don't use them more often than the instructions recommend. Also, black teens should *avoid* abrasives because their skin has a tendency to develop lighter or darker patches in the areas where they've used the abrasives.

Washing, even with antibacterial soaps or abrasives, isn't always enough to prevent pimples and doesn't do much to help acne. Occasionally, mild cases of acne can be cleared up by using medicated acne lotions and creams that are sold without prescription. If these medications and the washing routines we've described don't take care of your problem and you're really bothered by acne, you should see a dermatologist, a doctor who specializes in skin problems.

A lot of times, parents say, "Oh, it's not that bad," or "Leave it alone, you'll outgrow it." But if you take the time to explain to your parents how much your skin problems bother you, they'll probably listen. If your family doesn't have medical insurance or coverage that will pay for the dermatologist, you may find that your parents are concerned about the cost. Many families don't have money to spend on doctor's visits unless you're actually sick. If money is a problem, perhaps you can find some odd jobs to earn enough to pay for the dermatologist yourself. You might call some dermatologists; your family doctor or local medical association, which is listed in the yellow pages under "Physicians," can give you names of dermatologists in your area. Ask how much the doctor charges. Some doctors will let you work out a payment plan by which you give a little money each week until your bill is paid up.

What can a dermatologist do for you? Well, that depends. If blackheads are a problem, the doctor can use a device called a comedo extractor to remove the blackheads. The comedo extractor (*comedo* is the scientific term for blackhead) exerts pressure on the skin and causes the blackhead to pop out of the pore, thus unclogging the duct. The area around the blackhead may be a little red for a while, but unlike squeezing or "popping" your blackheads with your fingers, the comedo extractor won't cause scars. You should never pop your blackheads or pimples because you might wind up with permanent scars or pits. The extractor is used only on blackheads. Once you've got an actual pimple, using the extractor may cause more harm than good.

comedo (KOM-i-DOUGH)

The dermatologist can also prescribe drugs that are more effective than the medications you can buy without a doctor's prescription. For example, in certain cases, the dermatologist may prescribe a drug called tetracycline. Tetracycline kills germs and can fight the infections that often start in clogged pores and lead to acne. This drug also cuts down on the amount of sebum your oil glands produce. For some teens, tetracycline works miracles and completely cures their acne. However, you should only use it according to your doctor's orders because in some people it can cause problems, such as upset stomach and increased sensitivity to sunlight (sunburns). These and other side effects are usually pretty mild but you must follow your doctor's orders carefully.

If tetracycline doesn't work for you (and it *doesn't* work for everyone), your doctor may prescribe other treatments. He or she might, for instance, prescribe a gel or cream containing retinoic acid. This medication is effective when applied on the face, but it doesn't work on other areas, like your shoulders or back. For the first week or so, your face may look even worse, but then your skin will usually peel and look better. There are also other treatments a dermatologist can prescribe, so if you're troubled by skin problems, it may be worth your while to see a dermatologist.

Stretch Marks
Some boys and girls develop stretch marks, purplish or white lines on their skin, during puberty. This is fairly rare, but it does occur. It happens because the skin is stretched too much during rapid growth, and it loses its

tetracycline (TET-reh-SIGH-clean)
retinoic (reh-tin-OH-ic)

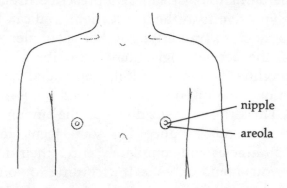

Illustration 16. The breast. In the center of each breast is a small raised part called the "nipple," which is surrounded by a ring of skin called the "areola."

elasticity, or stretchiness. (Other things, such as taking certain medications, being pregnant, or gaining a lot of weight can also cause stretch marks.) Many times these marks will fade or get less noticeable as a person gets older, but they may never disappear completely.

BREAST CHANGES

We usually think of breast change as something that happens to girls, because during puberty their breasts begin to grow and develop (as we explain in Chapter 6). Although boys' breasts don't change as dramatically as girls' do, there are certain changes in your breasts that you may notice at this time in your life. For one thing, the *areola*, the ring of colored flesh around your nipple, may get wider and darker in color (see Illustration 16). The nipple may also get a bit larger.

areola (ah-ree-OH-la)

You may notice that your breasts feel tender or sore. Many boys notice a flat, buttonlike bump under one or both nipples. If this happens to you and you don't know that it's perfectly normal, it can be a bit scary. As one man told us:

> I had these bumps under my nipples. I thought I had cancer or something.
>
> Harold, age 34

Even though these lumps can be uncomfortable, or even downright painful, they aren't anything to worry about. It's just a reaction to the new hormones your body is making. Eventually, the lumps and soreness will go away. It's perfectly normal and not a sign that you have cancer or any other disease. (Men, by the way, only rarely get cancer of the breast, and young boys almost *never* do.)

Out of every 100 boys between 50 and 85 of them will experience some swelling of the breasts as they go through puberty. In some boys, this swelling is more noticeable than in others. The swelling may be accompanied by soreness. There may also be lumps, of the type described above, under one or both breasts. This swelling can last from one year to a year and a half.

Although this, too, is a normal and natural change—and even though it happens to more than half of the boys going through puberty—boys really worry about it. Over the years, I've gotten a lot of questions about this in the question box in my class. Boys worry because they think they're going to start to grow breasts and turn into girls or something. One man who had quite a bit of breast swelling during puberty told us how he felt:

It was like I was growing breasts, and mine were even bigger than some of the girls'! I got teased about it all the time. I was really afraid that I was turning into a girl, that someone had made this big mistake and I really *was* a girl. I thought my penis was maybe going to fall off or something and I'd grow breasts and have to wear a bra. I'd heard all sorts of wild stories about boys who turned out to be women and had breasts *and* penises. But I didn't know anyone I could ask about it.

By the time I was in high school, my chest looked normal. My breasts had gone away. I wish I'd known that it was going to be okay because I really worried about it for a while.

Tom, age 40

You may also notice that your breasts are swelling, and you may have the same kind of worries Tom had. Relax—we promise, you won't turn into a girl! Within about a year to a year and a half, the swelling will go away. (If, like Tom, you've heard wild stories about boys who turned into women, you might want to read Chapter 7, page 175, to find out the real facts.)

VOICE CHANGES

Another change you may notice as you go through puberty is that your voice becomes lower and deeper. This happens because testosterone causes your *larynx*, or voice box (the part of your throat that contains your vocal cords), to grow larger. Your vocal cords get thicker and longer, and this changes the tone of your voice. Voice changes usually happen when a boy is about fourteen or fifteen, but they may happen earlier or later than this.

For some boys, this voice change happens without their really noticing it:

larynx (LARR-inks)

I didn't realize that my voice had changed, except that people stopped thinking I was my mom or my sister when I'd answer the phone.

Bill, age 19

For some boys, the change in their voices is more sudden and noticeable:

My throat was sore for about a month or so, kind of scratchy. I thought I just had some kind of sore throat. My voice was kind of froggy. I was always going ahem, ahem— you know, how you clear your throat. Afterward I noticed my voice was deeper than before.

Phil, age 17

Some boys experience what is called "cracking" of their voices as they're going through this voice change. They'll be talking in a normal voice and all of a sudden their voice will get very high and squeaky. A lot of boys found this cracking one of the most embarrassing things about going through puberty. As one man explained:

I'd finally get up my nerve to call a girl on the phone and ask her for a date. I'd say, "Hi, Susie," or whatever her name was, "this is John," and my voice would be just fine. I'd sound perfectly cool. Then I'd say, "Would you like to go to the movies?"—and right in the middle my voice would go all high and funny. It would sound like it was Minnie Mouse talking.

John, age 36

Another man said:

Really, it was the most embarrassing thing. It seemed like it happened about all the time. I'd try to control my voice and never get really excited or happy-sounding. Anytime I got nervous and excited, that's when it would happen. I tried not to get too emotional, but of course I did. I never really got control over it. Finally, after a year or maybe it was two years, it stopped happening.

> Tyrone, age 28

Your voice may change suddenly and dramatically or it may happen without your really noticing it. Like John and Tyrone, your voice may crack and you may feel embarrassed about it, although there's no real reason to be embarrassed, because people know it's just a part of growing up. Eventually, though, your voice will "settle down" and you'll find yourself sounding more adult.

PUBERTY IS NOT A DISEASE!

It usually takes an entire class period for us to cover the changes we've been talking about in this chapter. The kids in my class are curious about these things, and they often have a lot of questions. Most of them agree that knowing about things like sore or swollen breasts, pimples, stretch marks, and cracking voices helps you to deal with them if they happen to you. Still, hearing about all of them at once can be a bit overwhelming. As one boy put it:

> I'm not sure I'm exactly looking forward to all these things happening to me. Puberty is beginning to sound like some kind of disease!

Puberty definitely isn't a disease. The changes we've described in this chapter and in other parts of this book are natural and healthy. They're a normal part of growing up and becoming a man. Still, when we start focusing on things like perspiration, pimples, cracking voices, and so on, puberty can start to sound like just one hassle after another. By the end of the class in which we cover these things, I can see that some of the kids are starting to think that puberty sounds like more trouble than it's worth! So I tell them, "Hey, don't get discouraged!"

First of all, the problem things don't happen to everyone. Not everyone has pimples, a voice that cracks, or swollen, sore breasts. For most kids, the physical changes of puberty happen without any difficulties. And even for those who do have some problems, it's not such a big deal. So your voice cracks. Even if it's embarrassing, no one ever died of embarrassment.

Sometimes, spending a whole class period—or, in the case of this book, a whole chapter—on these problems can give you a distorted picture. It can make them loom larger or seem more important than they really are. So at the end of the class, I ask everyone to make a list of the five things they like best about going through puberty and growing up. Here are some of the things the boys in my classes have come up with.

more privileges	getting my braces off
getting to stay out later	getting a job
being more my own boss	dating
driving a car	getting into R-rated movies
new friends	having my body get stronger
new school	going to parties
more respect	having my own money
more allowance	joining the team in high school
making my own decisions (sometimes)	going to college
hanging out with the older guys	

Perhaps you'd like to take a few minutes to make a list of your own, to help yourself remember that puberty is a lot more than just pimples and perspiration!

CHAPTER 5

Ejaculation, Orgasms, Erections, Masturbation, and Wet Dreams

---

Way back in Chapter 1, we talked about ejaculation. We explained that when a man and a woman are having sexual intercourse, the man may ejaculate his sperm into the woman's vagina. When this happens, muscles in his genital area contract and sperm are pumped out of his testicles, through a hollow tube in the center of the penis, and out the opening in the center of the glans (the "tip" or "head") of his penis.

Men don't always ejaculate when they're having sex, but usually they do. A man or boy may ejaculate at other times too, even if he's not having sexual intercourse. In fact, boys usually have their first ejaculations just before their fourteenth birthdays, long before most of them have started having sexual intercourse. In this

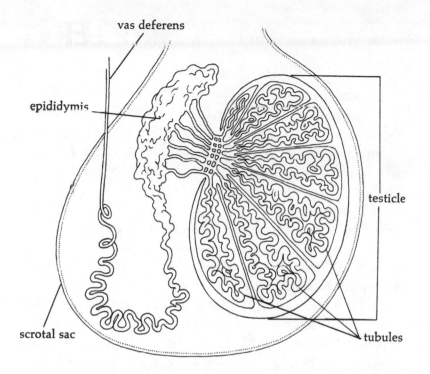

vas deferens

epididymis

testicle

scrotal sac

tubules

Illustration 17. Cross section of the scrotum. This drawing shows the inside of a scrotal sac. The sperm are made in the tubules, inside the testicle. Then they travel to the epididymis, where they ripen. From there, they move through the vas deferens, up into the main part of the body.

chapter, we'll talk about the things other than sexual intercourse that can cause you to ejaculate, and we'll also talk about your first ejaculation.

THE INSIDE STORY

In order to understand ejaculation, it helps to have some idea of how the sex organs on the inside of the body work. Illustration 17 shows a cross section of one of the scrotal sacs. (If this drawing looks a bit confusing to you or you've forgotten how cross-section drawings work, you might want to take another look at Illustration 5 on page 37.)

The Testicles

As you may recall, the testicles, or testes, rest inside the scrotum. Each testicle is made up of separate compartments. We couldn't draw small enough to get them all in this picture, but there are about two hundred and fifty of these little compartments in each testicle. Inside' each of these compartments are tiny, thread-like tubes called *tubules*, which are coiled up and packed tightly. If you unwound all the tubules in your testicles and stretched them out end to end, they'd stretch the length of several football fields.

During puberty, a boy begins to make sperm inside these tubules, and he continues to make fresh sperm through the rest of his life. Sperm production slows down a bit in old age, but until then, a male makes millions of sperm each day.

Sperm are alive. When they're fully mature, they look like tadpoles, with rounded bodies and tiny tails. Of course, real sperm are much smaller than the critter you

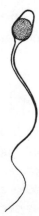

Illustration 18. A sperm

see in Illustration 18. In fact, it would take five hundred sperm, lined up end to end, to cover a distance of one inch. You can't even see a sperm unless you use a microscope.

The Epididymis

After the sperm are made, they travel from the tubules inside the testicle to the *epididymis*, a special compartment attached to the testicle. The epididymis is also composed of tiny tubes. It is here, inside these tubes, that the sperm ripen into mature sperm. It takes the sperm about four to six weeks to travel through the epididymis, during which time they complete their ripening.

The Vas Deferens

Once they're fully mature, the sperm are ready to travel out of the scrotal sac and up into the body, where they are stored until you ejaculate. To get from the scrotum to the main part of your body, the sperm travel through a tube called the *vas deferens* (also called the vas or sperm duct). You have two sperm ducts, one for each testicle. Each one is between fourteen and eighteen inches long. You can only see the bottom part of one vas in Illustration 17. But if you look at Illustration 19, you'll see that the rest of the vas runs up out of the scrotum and into the main part of your body.

Perhaps you've wondered why the testicles and scrotum hang down, outside and away from the main part of your body. As one boy in my class put it:

> Why do they dangle down there like that where they can get hit and knocked around? Why aren't they tucked up inside your body where they'd be safe?

epdidymis (eh-PIH-did-dih-mis)
vas (VAZ) *deferens* (DEAF-eh-wrens)

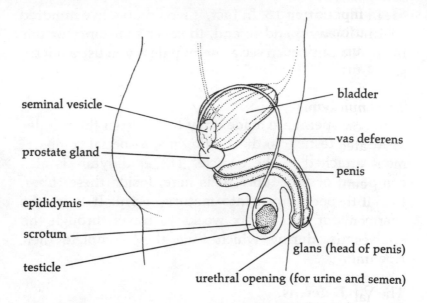

seminal vesicle

prostate gland

epididymis

scrotum

testicle

bladder

vas deferens

penis

glans (head of penis)

urethral opening (for urine and semen)

Illustration 19. Cross section of the sex organs on the inside of the male body

It's a good question, and there's a good answer. In order for your testicles to make sperm, they have to be at exactly the right temperature. The right temperature is a little *lower* than the temperature of the rest of your body. If your testicles were up inside your body, they'd get too hot to make sperm. So, instead, they hang down in the scrotal sac, away from your body. This way air can circulate around them and keep them cool. In cold weather or when you jump into a cold pool, the scrotum tightens up, bringing your testicles closer to your body for extra warmth. In hot weather, after a hot bath, or when you have a fever, the scrotum relaxes and hangs lower so that your testicles are farther away from your body and can stay cool.

The Ampulla

As you can see from Illustration 19, the vas deferens winds up over the bladder, the hollow, pouchlike organ where urine collects. Then the tube widens or flares out. The widened or flared-out portion of the tube is called the *ampulla*. The ampulla is a sort of "sperm storage tank" or reservoir, where sperm are kept until they're ejaculated.

The Seminal Vesicles

Just at the lower part of the ampulla, the *seminal vesicles* connect up to the vas. You have two seminal vesicles, but you can only see one in Illustration 19. *Seminal* refers to sperm, and *vesicle* means "little sac," so together the words mean "little sperm sac." The seminal vesicles got their name because scientists once thought that sperm were stored there until they were ejaculated. We now know that sperm are stored in the ampulla, but the name still sticks.

Even though they don't store sperm, the seminal vesicles have an important job. They make the white sticky fluid called *semen*, or seminal fluid, that spurts out of your penis when you ejaculate. Mixed in with this fluid are millions of sperm from your ampulla. But sperm are so tiny that they account for only about one-tenth of the teaspoon of milky fluid that comes out when you ejaculate. The other nine-tenths of your ejaculate is composed mostly of fluid from the seminal vesicles.

Semen

Semen is very powerful stuff. You know how during a game football players drink Gatorade, which is packed

ampulla (am-PUL-ah or am-POOL-ah)
seminal (SEM-eh-nul) *vesicles* (VES-eh-kuls)
semen (SEA-men)

full of sugar and vitamins, to give them an instant energy boost? Well, semen is like Gatorade for sperm. Just before ejaculation, the seminal vesicles release semen into the ampulla. The sperm are zapped by a shot of the sugar-rich semen, which gives them a big energy boost.

Until the seminal fluid mixes with the sperm, the sperm are sort of sluggish and slow-moving. They hardly move their tails. They don't even have enough energy to get around by themselves.

Luckily, the walls of the vas deferens have muscles that work something like the muscles in your throat. These muscles contract, and, with the help of tiny little hairs, they sweep the sperm up the tube of the vas deferens into the ampulla. Otherwise, the sluggish sperm would never get themselves out of the scrotum.

Once the sperm get a shot of semen, they start whipping their tails around like wild and moving all over the place. Sperm really need this energy boost. They have quite a long journey to make in order to get to the ovum and fertilize it. After the sperm and semen are ejaculated from the man's penis into the woman's vagina, the sperm have to travel to the top of the woman's vagina and through the narrow opening there that leads to her uterus. Then they have to travel the whole length of the woman's uterus and halfway up her fallopian tube in order to meet up with and fertilize the ovum. (Look back at Illustration 6, page 38, if you don't remember what these body parts look like.) And the sperm have to move quickly in order to get to the ovum while it's still nice and fresh. So the sperm are "running" the whole way.

Altogether it's only a distance of about six inches that the sperm have to travel, which doesn't sound like much. Remember, though, sperm are less than one five-hundredth of an inch long. Six inches to a sperm would be like four miles to a man. You'd certainly need an energy boost if you were going to run four miles at top speed!

The Prostate Gland

The prostate gland, which lies below the ampulla and seminal vesicles, is ring-shaped. A number of tubes, including the vas deferens, run through the center of this ring. The prostate gland also adds some fluid to the semen. When a man ejaculates, the prostate contracts and tightens up, squeezing on the vas. This helps push the sperm and the other seminal fluids (that is, the semen) into the tube in the center of the penis that is called the *urethra*.

The Urethra

The urethra is yet another tube. (Seems like you're just full of tubes, doesn't it?) As you can see from looking at Illustration 19, the urethra is in the center of the penis. It is cushioned by the soft, spongy tissue on the inside of the penis. The sperm and seminal fluid travel through the urethra and spurt out the opening in the center of the glans, or head, of the penis during ejaculation. Urine from the bladder also travels along the urethra when you urinate (pee). The tube from the bladder and the vas deferens both connect up with the urethra.

When I tell the kids in my class that urine and sperm both use the urethra to get out of the body, someone usually blurts out, "Oh, gross!" Even if no one says anything, I can see from their wrinkled-up noses and the looks on their faces that many kids think this sounds pretty disgusting.

prostate (PROS-tate)
urethra (you-REE-thra)

But, really, there's nothing gross or disgusting about it. Urine is just another liquid, and unless you have an infection, it doesn't have any disease-causing germs in it. Semen is perfectly clean too. Besides, sperm and urine can't travel through the urethra tube at the same time. When you're about to ejaculate, there's a valve at the bottom of the bladder that closes off so that urine can't get into the urethra when sperm is about to travel through there. Also, just before you ejaculate, two small glands in the area release a little bit of liquid into the urethra to flush it out and neutralize any acidy urine that might still be in there. (Sperm are sensitive to acids, so it's necessary to neutralize any acid in the urethra before the sperm travels through it.)

Even though I try to explain all this really carefully, I almost always get a question about it in the Everything You Ever Wanted to Know question box at the end of the class. Usually, the question has something to do with whether or not a man can urinate and ejaculate at the same time. Or, as one kid wrote, "Can a man piss inside a woman's vagina?"

I must admit, when I first got this question, I didn't quite understand it. I thought the kid who wrote it must have been putting me on. (Some kids in my classes do try to put me on, especially at the beginning of the year. They'll put questions in the box that have lots of so-called dirty words or are really gross, hoping to embarrass me when I read them out loud. But they soon give up on this because, as you may have guessed, I don't get embarrassed very easily, at least not by dirty words or questions about sex.)

At any rate, I finally figured out what the kid who wrote the question was getting at. He or she was wondering if a man could by accident urinate (piss) instead of ejaculate during sexual intercourse. Actually, when you think of how all those tubes are connected up, it's a pretty logical question. But the answer is no. When the penis gets stiff and hard—that is, when a male has an erection—that valve I mentioned earlier closes up. It seals off the bladder, and urine can't come through the urethra until the penis gets soft again.

EJACULATION AND ORGASM

When a male ejaculates, the muscles around the prostate gland, as well as the muscles in the penis and surrounding area, contract. These muscle contractions, or spasms, force most of the sperm out of the ampulla. The sperm and semen mix together and are pushed into the urethra. They're propelled along the urethra and come spurting out the opening in the glans, or tip, of the penis. The semen usually comes out in three or four spurts. In all, about a teaspoon or so of white, creamy, milky semen comes out of the penis during ejaculation.

The feeling that you get when all these muscles are contracting and semen is spurting out of your penis is called *orgasm*. It is possible to ejaculate without having an orgasm, but most of the time a male does have one when he ejaculates. Slang terms for having an orgasm include "coming," "climaxing," and "getting off."

It's a bit difficult to describe exactly what an orgasm feels like. For one thing, it feels different to different people. Also, the feeling of an orgasm may differ from one time to the next. Sometimes the orgasm may be really strong and involve not just the penis and other sex organs but the whole body. At other times, the orgasm may be less intense, and the feeling seems to center around the penis and the genital area.

orgasm (OR-gaz-um)

When a male is about to have an orgasm, his penis is stiff and erect. The skin on his scrotum gets tighter and thicker as the scrotum draws up close to his body. His heart starts beating harder and his breathing gets deeper and heavier. The skin on his face or chest or other parts of his body may get flushed and reddish in color. This is called the "sex flush." His nipples may become deeper in color and stiffer and may stand out more. The muscles around his anus may tighten up. A drop or two of clear or milky white fluid may appear at the tip of the penis. The opening in the head, or glans, of the penis may become more slit-like, and the glans may become a deeper, more purplish or red color.

As the orgasm is about to begin, the man may be aware of all these changes (the increase in heartbeat, the heavier breathing, the changes in the glans), but often the feeling is so intense that he is totally involved only in the feeling. The changes may happen without his being consciously aware of them.

During the actual orgasm, the muscles contract and the semen comes out in three or four spurts that usually happen within less than a second of one another. These spurts may be followed by a series of six to fifteen other muscle spasms. The whole orgasm normally lasts about ten seconds. The feeling is so intense, though, that it often seems longer.

After the orgasm, the heartbeat and breathing gradually return to normal. The testicles and scrotum loosen up. The penis gets soft again. All of this may take just a few seconds, or it may take a half hour or so. Afterward, men often feel really relaxed, and they may be sleepy. Other men are ready to have another orgasm right away. Usually, though, there's a period of time that must pass—anywhere from a few minutes to a half hour, several hours, or a day or so—before a man is ready to have another orgasm. Generally, the older a man gets, the more time it takes before he's ready to have another orgasm.

As we say, it's a little difficult to explain how an orgasm feels, but most people agree that it's a super good feeling. We asked the men we interviewed to describe it, and many said things like "great," "terrific," "beautiful," or other simple, one-word answers. Most had trouble putting it into words, saying things like, "There's just no words to describe it," or "It's not something you can explain." Some men, however, were able to give a description. One man gave a description that other men seemed to think was pretty good. Here's what he said:

> Well, it feels like there's a sort of neat sensation in my genitals and body that builds up and then goes off, a sort of wave of good sensual feeling throughout the whole body. The spurting part, when the semen is actually coming out, is a jerky kind of thing. It's not really all that great a feeling, but the waves of the sensual feeling are timed with pulses of the spurt, which does feel great. Afterward, I feel tingling and then relaxed all over.
>
> Will, age 46

ERECTIONS

Before a male has an ejaculation or an orgasm, his penis gets stiff and hard, or at least semi-hard (halfway, or a little bit, hard). As you may recall from Chapter 1, this is called having an erection, or, in slang terms, a "boner" or a "hard-on." (You don't have an ejaculation every time you have an erection, however, just sometimes.)

During an erection, the blood passageways in the spongy tissue on the inside of the penis fill with blood.

This causes the penis to get stiff and hard and stand out from the body. Of course, there's always *some* blood inside your penis, just as there's always some blood in every part of your body. Our hearts are continually pumping blood throughout our bodies, and this flow of blood helps keep each part of us healthy and strong. But when the penis is erect there's more blood than usual in it. The muscles at the base of the penis tighten up and close off the passageways that normally allow blood to flow out of the penis, trapping the blood and causing the penis to swell and become larger and harder.

An erection can happen very quickly. In just a few seconds, the penis may go from being completely soft and floppy to being quite hard. Or an erection may happen more slowly and gradually. Sometimes the penis gets *really* hard and stiff. At other times, the penis may get only semi-hard.

When the penis gets erect, it also gets longer and wider. It may get darker in color. The scrotum and testicles may pull up tighter and closer to the body. The blood vessels (blood passageways) on the surface of the penis may bulge out, and the skin covering the blood vessels may turn bluish or darker in color.

Some penises are quite straight when they are erect, but many are slightly curved or bent. Sometimes the erect penis stands out at a right angle from the body, but usually it points upward. It may even stick practically straight up (see Illustration 20).

Erections happen for all sorts of reasons. Stroking or touching the penis or the scrotum often causes an erection. The friction of your pants rubbing against your penis can cause one. Sometimes the penis becomes erect even though it has not been touched or rubbed. At times, a male may have an erection when he needs to urinate, or he may wake up in the morning with an erection.

Thinking "sexy" thoughts—that is, thinking about having sex, about being sexual, about your sex organs, or just about sex in general—may cause an erection. But sometimes males have erections even though they are not thinking about sex at all. Getting nervous or excited about something can cause an erection. Warm, nice feelings can cause one. In fact, erections sometimes happen when you are not thinking about anything in particular.

Males have erections, from time to time, throughout their whole lives. Even tiny babies have erections. Many boys find that once they start puberty, they have erections more frequently than they did before. They often have what we call "spontaneous erections." Spontaneous erections happen spontaneously—that is, "all by themselves"—even though the penis has not been stroked or touched. They can happen anywhere, at any

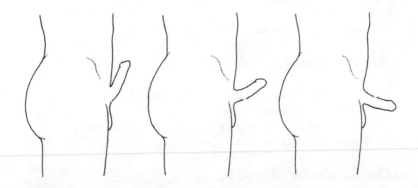

Illustration 20. Erections. The erect penis may stick out at various angles or may stand practically straight up.

spontaneous (spon-TAY-knee-us)

time. As we said, they may happen when you are thinking about sex or girls, when you get excited or nervous, or even when you are not feeling any particular way or thinking about anything in particular.

Not all boys notice that they start to have more erections than ever before as they are going through puberty. But many boys do. It is normal if you do and normal if you don't.

Boys who do have erections more frequently during puberty may have them quite often or only once in a while. The boys and men we interviewed for this book were very different in this way. Some rarely, if ever, had spontaneous erections. Others had them once a month; others once or twice a week. Still others had erections ten or twelve times a day.

The boys and men we talked to were often embarrassed when they had spontaneous erections. One boy in my class told a story that went something like this:

I was on the beach wearing my BVs [a bikini kind of bathing suit made out of thin, nylon material], and I saw this really curvy girl lying on her towel. My penis got hard and I had to run into the ocean so no one would see.

Another said:

Yeah, I get erections sometimes when I'm out running. That's how come I always wear a pair of gym shorts over my sweat pants. You get a hard-on and it sticks out like a tent pole in those baggy sweats.

One man remembered how it was for him:

It would happen any old time. I'd be at school, standing in the hall or something, and bingo, I'd have a hard-on. I'd shuffle my school books around and try and hold them in front of me so no one could see. It was really embarrassing.

Joe, age 32

Many told stories about getting erections when they had to get up in front of the class:

> I had to give a speech one time in public-speaking class. I had this really funny speech, and I'm standing there doing it and I get this big hard-on. I didn't know if everyone was laughing at my speech or at my hard-on.
>
> Tyrone, age 28

If you start to notice that you're having more erections as you're going through puberty, it helps to know that it's perfectly normal, that other boys are experiencing the same thing, and that your erections probably aren't as noticeable to other people as they are to you.

ONCE YOU HAVE AN ERECTION

Once you have an erection, one of two things will happen. First of all, the erection may go away all by itself. It may take a few seconds, a few minutes, or even a half hour or so before your penis is completely soft again. But after a while the muscles at the base of your penis will relax, allowing the extra blood that was trapped in the penis to flow back out so that the penis becomes soft and floppy again.

The second thing that can happen is that you will ejaculate and/or have an orgasm, after which the muscles at the base of the penis will relax and the penis will become soft again. As we explained, one thing that can cause a male to have an orgasm and to ejaculate is sexual intercourse. During sexual intercourse, the man puts his erect (or at least semi-erect) penis into the woman's vagina. As you may recall from Chapter 1, the vagina is a hollow organ. Normally, the vagina is like a collapsed balloon with no air in it; but it is very expandable, so the penis can fit right in there (see Illustration 21). The vagina fits snugly and tightly around

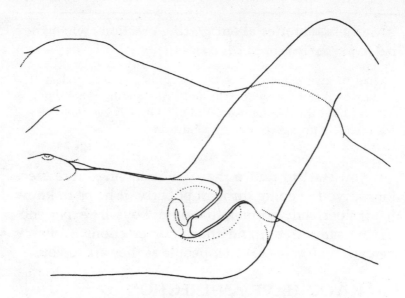

Illustration 21. Penis in vagina

the penis. During intercourse, a man moves his penis around in the vagina, which stimulates the nerves in the penis. When the penis is sufficiently stimulated, the man usually ejaculates. It's possible to ejaculate without having an orgasm. It's also possible to have an orgasm without ejaculating. But usually when a man is having sexual intercourse, he both ejaculates *and* has an orgasm. Soon afterward, his penis becomes soft again.

MASTURBATION

Another thing that can cause a male to ejaculate and/or have an orgasm is masturbation. *Masturbation* means "deliberate touching or stroking of the sex organs." Slang terms for masturbating include "jacking off," "playing with yourself," "beating your meat," "doing

masturbation (mass-tur-BAY-shun)

it," and "pulling the joystick." If a man or boy masturbates long enough, he usually has an orgasm. He doesn't always have an orgasm when he masturbates; sometimes he stops masturbating before he gets to that point. Or, if he's just recently had an orgasm and starts masturbating again, he may not be able to have another one until his body has had a chance to rest up. A little while after he has had an orgasm, his penis becomes soft again. Even if he masturbates and doesn't have an orgasm, his erection will still go away after a while.

A boy may masturbate to the point of orgasm before he begins to go through puberty, but he doesn't start ejaculating until he starts making sperm in his testicles. Many boys don't masturbate until they start puberty and begin making sperm. Such boys may find that they have their first orgasm at the same time that they have their first ejaculation.

The first ejaculation usually happens around the age of thirteen or fourteen. But some boys ejaculate before this, and others don't have ejaculations until they're fifteen and older. For some boys, the first ejaculation happens as a result of masturbating. For others, the first ejaculation happens in their sleep. This is called having a wet dream. We'll explain more about wet dreams later in this chapter, but for now we want to talk more about masturbation. Kids usually have lots of questions about masturbation, and here are answers to some of those questions.

Do most boys masturbate?
Yes, most boys (and men, too) masturbate. Not all do, though. It's normal if you do and normal if you don't.

Some men start to masturbate when they're kids and continue throughout their lives. Some start during

masturbates (MASS-tur-baits)

puberty. Some don't start until they're older. And there are some who never masturbate.

People sometimes think that the only men who masturbate are those who haven't started having sexual intercourse yet. They get the idea that once you start having sex, you stop masturbating. Not true. Many married men and also unmarried men, even if they're having sexual intercourse regularly, still masturbate.

Do girls masturbate?
Yes, girls and women also masturbate. Women don't, of course, ejaculate sperm like men do, but their genitals may feel very wet when they masturbate. This is because glands in the vulva and vagina give off fluids when a female becomes sexually aroused. Some women's glands produce a sudden gush of fluid just as they're having an orgasm, but this is not an ejaculation of the type men have.

According to studies done by sex researchers, boys are more likely to masturbate than girls. But many of these studies were done ten or twenty years ago. Today, it's considered more acceptable for girls to know about and talk about their bodies, so many experts feel that nowadays the number of girls who masturbate (or are willing to admit that they masturbate) may be much higher.

How often do boys masturbate?
This depends on the boy. Some masturbate several times a day; some once or twice a day; some once or twice a week. Some boys masturbate more often or less often than this, and some never masturbate.

Is masturbation bad for you?
No, masturbation is not in any way harmful. Back in your grandmother and grandfather's day, people

thought that all sorts of horrible things would happen if you masturbated. Masturbation was supposed to cause warts on your nose, hair to grow on the palms of your hands, pale skin, pimples, wet and clammy hands, blindness, softening of the brain, idiocy, and insanity (to mention just a few problems). Nowadays we know that none of these things is true. (If they were, there would be an awful lot of blind, insane idiots around.)

Even though people no longer believe these old stories, the idea that masturbation might be harmful or just not good for you still lingers on. Some people think that masturbating too much will cause you to "run out of" or "use up" all your sperm. But, as you know from reading this book, your body is constantly making millions of new sperm each day. There's just no way you could run out. Other people think that masturbating too much will somehow hurt your penis or sex organs. Again, this isn't true. If you masturbate and ejaculate a whole lot, your penis might get sore from all the rubbing, but other than this soreness, masturbating cannot hurt your body. In fact, it's just not possible for you to masturbate and ejaculate too much. Your body sets its own limits. If a boy is masturbating a great deal, after a while his penis just won't get erect anymore. He'll have to rest for a while before he can get an erection again.

Is it all right to imagine things when you masturbate?
Many people like to imagine things that make them feel more excited as they are masturbating. Imagining or pretending that something is happening is called daydreaming or fantasizing. We daydream and fantasize about all sorts of things. We might, for instance, daydream about being a major league football player or a rock star. When our daydreams are about sexual things, we call them sexual fantasies. Almost everyone has sex-

ual fantasies. We may have them while we're masturbating and at other times too. Sexual fantasies are a rich and varied way of experimenting with your sexual self. Sometimes, the things we fantasize about are things we might actually like to do someday; other times we fantasize about things that we'd feel embarrassed or even bad about if we actually did them.

Some people worry that there might be something weird about their sexual fantasies. If you've ever been concerned about this, you can relax. Human beings (both males *and* females) have sexual fantasies about all sorts of things. If you think you're the only one who's ever had a particular fantasy—you're wrong. We guarantee that there are plenty of other people who've had almost the exact same fantasy.

Can masturbation affect your athletic performance?
In general, masturbating won't affect your athletic ability. Some athletic coaches think that it's a good idea for boys to masturbate before a big game. Masturbating is a way of relieving tension and is very relaxing. But there are some coaches who think that athletes perform better when they're somewhat tense and not completely relaxed, so they tell their teams to lay off masturbating or having sexual intercourse for a few days before a big game. If you're an athlete, you'll have to decide for yourself what works best for you.

Will masturbating a lot when you're young affect your sex life when you're older?
Some people think that if you masturbate a whole lot when you're young, you'll learn to like it so much that you won't enjoy sexual intercourse as much when you're older. This isn't true. In fact, most experts agree that masturbating is a way of rehearsing for your adult

sex life. By masturbating, you learn how your own body responds and what gives you the most pleasure. When you do begin to have sex, you are knowledgeable about what you like, about what "turns you on." If you know this about yourself, it's that much easier to tell your sex partner what you like and/or don't like and how your partner can help increase your sexual pleasure.

It is true that many men find that they have more physically intense orgasms from masturbation than from intercourse. (This doesn't necessarily mean that they *like* masturbation more than intercourse, because intercourse involves touching, holding, and being intimate with another person. That makes it a very different kind of experience than masturbating.) However, other men find that the orgasms they experience during intercourse are more intense than those they have during masturbation. Still others don't find any difference in intensity.

As you grow older, you may find that masturbating provides the most intense orgasms, that sexual intercourse does, or that both things provide equally intense orgasms. Regardless, how much or how little you masturbate when you're young won't have anything to do with what type of orgasms are most intense for you when you're an adult.

Is masturbation "sinful" or morally wrong?
One person's idea of what's "sinful" or morally wrong may be quite different from another person's. Nowadays, most people do not think masturbation is morally wrong or sinful, and personally, we go along with that point of view. In the past, many religions held that masturbation was a sin, and although many religious leaders no longer feel this way, some still do. The Cath-

olic religion's official point of view holds that masturbation is a sin. This doesn't mean, however, that all Catholics or even all Catholic priests and church leaders feel this way.

People who consider masturbation a sin often point to the story of Onan in the Bible (Genesis, Chapter 3, verses 9-10), in which Onan is punished by God for "spilling his seed on the ground." They feel that the story of Onan is a story about masturbation (masturbation used to be called onanism), and that it shows that God disapproves of masturbation. Others don't feel that this is what the story of Onan is all about. People who think masturbation is sinful usually feel that God approves of a man ejaculating only during intercourse with his wife, and that a man should practice enough self-control so that he only ejaculates under those circumstances.

As we said, what one person thinks is sinful or morally wrong may be different from what another person thinks. It's an individual thing, something you'll have to decide for yourself. If you're bothered by the notion that masturbation may be sinful or morally wrong, perhaps you should talk with your minister, priest, or religious leader, or maybe you'll find some of the publications we've listed in the back of this book helpful (see For Further Reading, pages 207–211).

Is it weird for a boy to masturbate with other boys?
Some boys have their first experience with masturbation by watching other boys, and it's not unusual for groups of boys to masturbate together. Some boys also experiment with masturbation by touching another boy's penis, by masturbating another boy to the point of orgasm, or by letting another boy masturbate them. Boys who do this often worry about whether this is

weird. Sometimes they think that this means that they are homosexual.

Homosexuals are people who prefer to have sexual contacts with people who are the same sex as they are. Most adults in our society are heterosexuals, which means that they prefer to have sexual experiences with people of the opposite sex. We'll talk more about homosexuality in Chapter 7, but for now you should know that masturbating with other boys, masturbating another boy, or thinking about doing either of these things does not mean you are a homosexual. Many boys engage in some form of what we call "sex play" with other boys as they're growing up, just as some girls engage in sex play with other girls, and some kids engage in sex play with members of the opposite sex as they're growing up. None of these sexual experiences is at all weird in the sense of being uncommon or unusual. If you've had such experiences and have wondered about them or felt uncomfortable, be sure to read Chapter 7, where we talk more about these things.

Do married people masturbate?
Yes, many people masturbate even though they have regular sex partners. They may masturbate privately (that is, when they're alone), or they may include masturbation as part of their sex lives with each other. They may masturbate before they have intercourse as a way of "warming up" or getting ready. Or they may masturbate instead of having intercourse, especially if the couple doesn't want to take the risk of the woman getting pregnant. (Unless a man ejaculates in the vagina or near the opening of the vagina, the sperm can't get

homosexual (hoe-moe-SEK-shoo-well)
heterosexual (HET-er-oh-SEK-shoo-well)
homosexuality (hoe-moe-sek-shoo-WAL-ity)

into her uterus and tubes to fertilize the ovum.) If a man ejaculates before the woman has an orgasm, masturbation can be a way for her to have an orgasm even though his penis is no longer erect and they can't continue having intercourse.

If a boy doesn't masturbate or have sexual intercourse, what happens to all the sperm?
If a boy doesn't ejaculate, either through masturbation or intercourse, one of two things may happen. As the ampulla becomes full, the sperm may simply dribble into the urethra, be mixed in with his urine, and be eliminated from his body when he urinates. Or he may have a wet dream.

WET DREAMS

As we explained earlier in this chapter, boys sometimes ejaculate while they're asleep. A common term for this is "having a wet dream." The scientific name for wet dreams is nocturnal emissions. *Nocturnal* means "during the night," and *emissions* are things that are "emitted" or "sent forth." So nocturnal emissions are ejaculations (sperm emitted or sent forth) at night.

It's possible for a grown man to have a wet dream, but they are much more common among boys going through puberty. Not all boys have wet dreams at this time in their lives, but many do. A boy who masturbates regularly is less likely to have a wet dream than one who never or only rarely masturbates. However, even boys who masturbate may have wet dreams fairly often.

Many boys have their first ejaculation during a wet dream. If you don't know about wet dreams and haven't

nocturnal (nok-TUR-nul)
emissions (e-MISH-uns)

been prepared for the fact that it may happen to you, a wet dream can be a confusing experience. Many boys thought they'd wet their beds or were bleeding or something until they realized that the fluid was milky white, not like blood or urine. As one man we interviewed explained:

> I'm what?—sixty-seven years old—so this is over fifty years ago, but I still remember my first wet dream like it was yesterday. Nobody told me anything about anything. So I woke up in the middle of the night. There's this wet, sticky stuff all over my belly. I thought, jeez, I wet my bed—at my age! I was thirteen or fourteen at the time.
>
> So a few days, maybe a week later, it happens again. Only now I pay more attention, and it's not piss [urine]. It's white and thick like a lotion or cream, sticky. I think I've got some kind of sickness. It keeps happening, so finally I tell my mother. She says if I control myself and don't think about "such things," it won't happen. I have no idea what she's talking about—control myself from what? Don't think about what things? I wasn't thinking about anything. I was asleep.
>
> Charlie, age 67

Even if you know about wet dreams beforehand, they can be a surprising experience, as one boy told me after class one day:

> My mom and dad had told me all about this kind of stuff ever since I was a kid. Still, it was a surprise the first time. Everything was hazy, but there was this wetness on my pajamas, and for a while I couldn't figure things out. I was only half awake. Then as I woke up more, I thought, "Oh, yeah, this is what Mom had said about."

Regardless of whether or not you know about wet dreams beforehand, you may feel embarrassed if you have one. One of the films I use in my sex-education classes, a film called *Am I Normal?*, deals with one young boy's experience as he's going through puberty. In one scene, the boy wakes up after having had a wet dream. He's so embarrassed that he takes off his pajamas and the sheets off his bed and sneaks down the hall to the bathroom. He turns the water on in the sink and pours a glass of water over his bedclothes and stuffs them in the laundry hamper. His mom hears him and calls out, "Is that you, honey? Is there anything wrong?"

"Nothing, Mom. . . . Oh, by the way, Mom, I forgot to tell you . . . I spilled water all over my bed," he nervously explains. "I guess I'm going to have to put my sheets in the hamper."

The boys in my class always get a big laugh out of this scene, probably because many of them have felt the same kind of embarrassment. But wet dreams aren't anything to be embarrassed about. They're a natural and normal thing, just another part of growing up.

After the class in which I show this film, there are usually at least a couple of questions about wet dreams in the Everything You Ever Wanted to Know question box. Two questions that come up over and over again are, "Do wet dreams only happen at night?" and "Do they only happen when you're asleep?" The answer is that wet dreams could happen anytime you're asleep. If you took a nap during the day, it would be possible for you to have a wet dream. But wet dreams only happen when you're asleep. You don't ejaculate when you're awake unless you decide to ejaculate. You might have a spontaneous erection, an erection that happens all by itself, but you won't have an ejaculation unless you deliberately decide to have one by masturbating or by having sexual intercourse.

The kids in my class also want to know why they're called *wet dreams*. "Do they only happen if you're having a dream?" "Do you have to be having a sexy dream?" they ask. The fact of the matter is that everyone dreams when he or she is asleep. Even if you don't remember doing so, you've been having dreams (a fact scientists have discovered by studying the electrical patterns in the brains of sleeping people). But the term *wet dream* doesn't mean that you dream during a nocturnal emission. It just refers to the fact that wet dreams happen when you're asleep, or at least half asleep. You may have been having a "sexy dream" during your nocturnal emission. Many boys who awake to find that they have ejaculated recall that their dream was about something sexual. But you may have a wet dream even if you haven't been having a sexual dream.

By the way, Charlie's mother was wrong. A boy can't stop himself from having wet dreams. They're just something that happens. In fact, wet dreams, like masturbation, are part of your body's way of emptying out the ampulla and making way for new sperm.

After you've read this far in the book, you've probably learned just about everything you've ever wanted to know about what happens to a boy's body during puberty. But we haven't talked very much about what happens to *girls'* bodies. So in the next chapter, we'll learn about girls and puberty.

CHAPTER 6

Girls and Puberty

Each year my daughter, Area, and I get together with a bunch of our friends and rent a houseboat. We spend a week cruising up and down the California Delta, the series of rivers that lead into the San Francisco Bay. We swim and fish and dig for clams and have mud fights and lie around in the sun and have a wonderful time just doing nothing at all. It's pretty much the same group of us every year. All of the adults are single mothers or single fathers, and we all have daughters about the same age. The girls went to grade school together. In fact, that's how we adults got to know one another in the first place.

We've been getting together like this for a number of years. Our daughters are teenagers now, and they go to different schools. Even though we've all gone our separate ways since the girls were little—some of us have even moved to different cities or towns—we still get together every year for this houseboat cruise.

Well, one year it just so happened that Area and I were putting the finishing touches on the book about girls and puberty when it came time for our annual cruise. Because we were going to spend a week on board a boat with six teenage girls, I figured that I'd take the rough draft of the book along and try to talk the girls into reading through the various chapters and making comments or suggestions. The girls were all about the same age, but they were in various stages of puberty. I thought that the more developed ones might be interested in the later chapters and that the girls who weren't so developed might want to read the earlier chapters.

I was wrong. All the girls wanted to read the same chapter—the one about boys. They couldn't have cared less about the rest of the book! They grabbed that chapter and went giggling off to the roof of the houseboat with their towels and suntan lotion and read it together. Later on, some of the girls read other chapters, but the big hit was definitely the chapter about boys.

I think their reaction was a pretty normal one. As we're going through puberty, we usually get at least some information about what's happening to our own bodies, if not from our parents and teachers then from our friends. A lot of times, though, parents and teachers don't tell us about what's happening to the opposite sex. They may feel that we just don't need to know this information, or that telling us will make us "too interested" in the opposite sex or will make us want to rush out and have sexual intercourse. Our friends may not know much more about this subject than we do.

All this makes it difficult for us to find out what's going on, and not knowing how puberty happens in the opposite sex can make everything seem a lot more confusing and mysterious than it needs to be. So in this

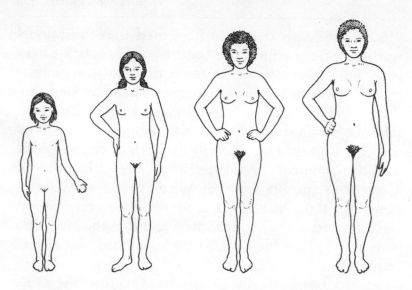

Illustration 22. Puberty in girls. As a girl goes through puberty, her hips get wider. Fat tissue begins to grow around her hips, thighs, and buttocks, giving her body a curvier shape. Her breasts begin to swell, and soft nests of hair begin to grow under her arms and on her genitals.

chapter, we'll be talking about how puberty happens in girls' bodies. If you're like most boys, you'll probably be pretty curious about this. (In fact, we wouldn't be surprised if this was the first chapter you turned to in this book.)

SIMILARITIES AND DIFFERENCES

As you can see from Illustration 22, girls' bodies also change quite a bit as they go through puberty. In some ways, puberty in girls is similar to puberty in boys. Both sexes undergo a growth spurt and a change in the general shape of their body. Both boys and girls begin to grow pubic hair. Boys start to make sperm for the first time, and girls produce their first ripe ova. The genital organs of both sexes begin to develop. Both boys and girls begin to perspire more, to take on adult body odors, and to get pimples at this time in their lives.

But boys and girls are different, so puberty happens a bit differently in girls than in boys. Some of the things that happen to boys don't happen to girls. For instance, girls don't experience the same lowering and deepening of the voice that boys do. Also, there are things that happen to girls that don't happen to boys, such as development of the breasts.

Even though boys and girls don't go through the exact same physical changes during puberty, their feelings about their body changes and their emotional reactions to growing up are, as we shall see, very similar. Let's start with the physical changes.

THE GROWTH SPURT

Like boys, girls go through a growth spurt during puberty and start to grow taller at a faster rate. The girls' growth spurt usually happens about two years before the boys' growth spurt. So at the age of eleven or twelve, girls often grow taller than the boys their age. However, a couple of years later, when the boys begin their growth spurt, they start to catch up to the girls. The boys' growth spurt lasts longer than the girls', and boys tend to add more inches during this time, so boys usually end up being taller than girls. Of course, there are some girls who will always be taller than most of the boys. But often a girl who is taller than the boys in her class when she's eleven or twelve will find that the boys have caught up by the age of thirteen or fourteen.

CHANGING SHAPE

The general shape, or contour, of a girl's body also changes as she goes through puberty. Her hips get wider, and fat tissue grows around the hips, buttocks, and thighs. This gives her body a curvier, rounder, more "womanly" shape.

PUBIC HAIR

Girls, too, begin to grow hair during puberty. In girls, the pubic hair begins to grow on the vulva. For some girls, this is the first change they notice as they begin puberty.

Just as doctors have divided the growth of the male sex organs into five stages, so they've divided the development of female pubic hair into five stages, shown in Illustration 23. Stage 1 is the childhood stage. It begins at birth and continues until a girl reaches Stage 2. A girl doesn't have any pubic hair during Stage 1. Stage 2 starts when the first curly pubic hairs appear, which is generally around the age of eleven, although it can happen earlier or later.

During Stage 3, the pubic hairs get darker and curlier. There are more of them, and they cover a wider area. Girls usually reach Stage 3 around the age of twelve. In Stage 4, which usually occurs between the ages of twelve and thirteen, the pubic hair gets still thicker and curlier and covers an even wider area.

Stage 5 is the adult stage. The pubic hair grows in an upside-down triangle pattern. In some women, the pubic hair grows up toward the belly button or out toward the thighs. The typical girl reaches this stage around the age of fourteen.

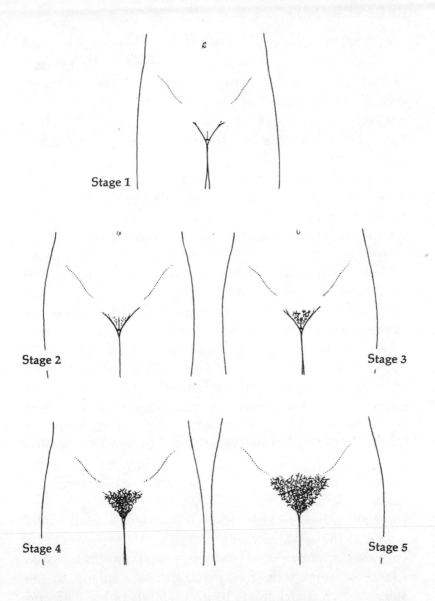

Illustration 23. The five stages of a girl's pubic hair growth

BREASTS

You may have heard all sorts of slang words used to refer to a girl's breasts—"boobs," "boobies," "knockers," "melons," "jugs," "tits," "titties," or whatever. Regardless of what you call them, you've probably noticed that they grow larger during puberty. Doctors have divided female breast development into the five stages shown in Illustration 24.

Stage 1 is the childhood stage. The breasts have not yet begun to develop. Stage 2 is the beginning of breast development. A small, buttonlike mound, similar to the ones some boys develop, forms under each nipple. The breasts may be sore or tender or even downright painful, especially if they're hit. The nipple gets larger, and the areola gets wider. Both the nipple and areola get darker in color, and the buttonlike mound underneath causes them to swell and stand out from the chest more. Most girls reach Stage 2 around the age of eleven.

In Stages 3 and 4, the breasts continue to get larger, rounder, and fuller, and they stand out from the chest more. The average girl reaches Stage 3 when she's about twelve, and Stage 4 when she's about thirteen. Girls stay in Stage 4 of breast development for a while, and most don't reach Stage 5 until they are about fifteen. Of course, not all girls are average, so some will reach these stages when they're a bit younger, and some when they're a bit older. Stage 5 is the adult stage.

Just as the age at which a boy starts to go through the various stages of puberty doesn't have anything to do with how quickly he goes through those stages, so the age at which a girl starts to go through pubic hair and breast development doesn't have anything to do with how quickly she gets to the adult stage. Some early starters develop quickly and some slowly; the same

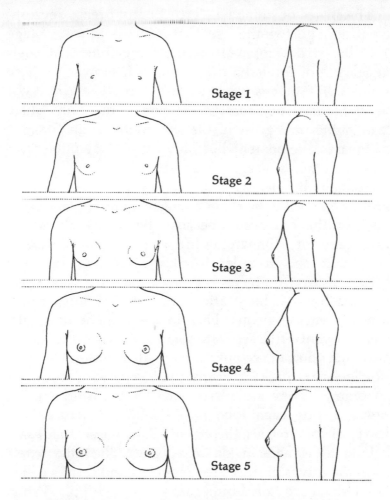

Illustration 24. The five stages of breast development

thing happens with late starters. There are some girls who develop *very* quickly. Such girls may start Stage 2 and reach Stage 3 within six months. After another six months, they've reached Stage 5. Other girls take six or more years to go from Stage 2 to Stage 5. The typical girl takes about four years to go from Stage 2 to Stage 5.

The stages of pubic hair growth and breast development may go together, so that a girl is in, say, Stage 3 of breast development at the same time that she's in Stage 3 of pubic hair development. However, these stages don't always coincide. For example, a girl might be in Stage 3 of breast development but only Stage 2 of pubic hair growth. Or she might be in Stage 4 of breast development but only Stage 2 of pubic hair growth.

You may be curious as to why a girl's breasts start to grow larger. Like the other changes that happen during puberty, this one occurs because the girl's body is getting ready for a time in her life when she may decide to have children. In order to understand why a girl's breasts grow, you have to know what's happening inside her breasts. Illustration 25 shows the inside of a grown woman's breast. Each breast is made up of fifteen to twenty-five separate compartments called *lobes*, although you can see only three of them in this picture. The lobes are packed together like separate sections of an orange. They are surrounded by a cushion of fat tissue. Inside each lobe is a treelike structure. The leaves of this tree are the *alveoli*. When a woman has a baby, milk is made inside these leaves. The milk travels from the leaves, through the branches and trunks of the tree (which are called milk ducts), to the nipple. When a mother breast-feeds, the baby sucks on the nipple and milk comes out.

As a girl begins puberty, she starts to develop milk ducts, alveoli, and fat tissue to cushion these milk-producing organs. Her breasts aren't yet ready to make milk and won't be until after she has had a baby. But

alveoli (al-vee-OH-lie)

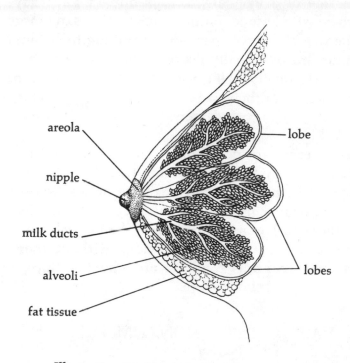

areola

nipple

milk ducts

alveoli

fat tissue

lobe

lobes

Illustration 25. Cross section of a woman's breast

her body is getting ready for this possibility, which is why her breasts grow larger.

Feelings about Developing Breasts
Just as some boys worry about whether their penis is "big enough," so girls often worry about the size of their breasts. Many girls (and women, too) wish their breasts were larger. Women with large breasts are supposed to be more feminine, more womanly, or sexier than smaller-breasted women. At least, that's the idea that you might get from all the big-breasted, glamorous women we see in advertisements, on TV, and in movies.

But the size of a woman's breasts doesn't have any-thing to do with how feminine or sexual she is, no more than the size of a man's penis has anything to do with how masculine or sexually powerful he is. Like a penis, breasts work equally well (produce the same amount of milk) regardless of their size.

Bras
As their breasts are developing, many girls begin to wear bras. Some wear them so that their breasts don't jiggle around when they run or dance or play sports, which can be uncomfortable. The support the bra gives makes them feel more comfortable. Some girls wear bras because they feel self-conscious without them. Others don't wear bras at all. It's an individual thing, a matter of personal choice.

BODY HAIR, PERSPIRATION, PIMPLES, AND OTHER CHANGES

Girls also grow new hair on their arms and legs during puberty, although such body hair isn't usually as thick as it is on boys. Some girls shave the hair on their legs with razors or use chemical hair removers to get rid of the hair. Others don't bother. Again, this is an indi-vidual thing, a matter of personal choice.

Underarm hair also develops during puberty, and some girls shave this hair. Perspiration and oil glands in the genital area, the underarms, the face, neck, shoul-ders, and back also become more active in girls during puberty, just as they do in boys. Some girls choose to use underarm deodorants; others don't. Some women use the deodorant sprays made for the vulvar and vaginal area. But these sprays can cause irritations, so we don't think they're a good idea.

Beginning with puberty, a girl's genitals may have a moister feeling due to the change in the oil and sweat glands in this area.

Pimples, acne, and stretch marks may be a problem for girls, just as they are for some boys.

THE GENITALS

A boy's scrotum and penis develop and change during puberty, and a girl's genital organs also change in appearance. Pubic hair grows on the mons and outer lips. The mons, the outer lips, and the inner lips get fatter and fleshier. The lips get larger, more wrinkly, and darker in color. The clitoris, urinary opening, and vaginal opening get a bit larger too.

The Hymen

A girl's *hymen* also gets thicker and more noticeable during puberty. The hymen is a thin piece of skin tissue that lies just inside the vaginal opening. Slang terms for it are "cherry" or "maidenhead."

The hymen looks different in different women. In some, it may be just a thin fringe of skin around the edges of the opening to the vagina. It may stretch across the opening and have one or more holes in it. Illustration 26 shows a close-up of different women's vaginal openings and some of the ways a hymen may look.

In young girls, the hymen may not be very noticeable. During puberty, it gets thicker, more rigid, and more noticeable. Not every female has a hymen, though. Some women are simply born without one. Other women's hymens are so torn or stretched that it's hard to see them.

hymen (HI-men)

As strange as it seems, this tiny piece of skin was once considered *very* important by many people. People used to think that all women had the kind of hymen that stretches all the way across the vaginal opening. They thought that the only way a hymen could be stretched or torn was if a man put his penis inside a woman's vagina while they were having sex. Today, we know this isn't true. For one thing, not all women have a hymen. Of those that do, not all have the kind that stretches all the way across the vaginal opening. Some have a hymen that is just a fringe of tissue around the edges of the vaginal opening; some have such a small, thin one that it is hardly noticeable. Also, hymens can get stretched or torn in a number of ways. Horseback riding, doing a split, falling off a bike—any stretching movement can tear the hymen. Whether or not a woman has a hymen has nothing to do with whether or not she has had sex with a man. In fact, some women have sexual intercourse quite a number of times without their hymen stretching or tearing at all.

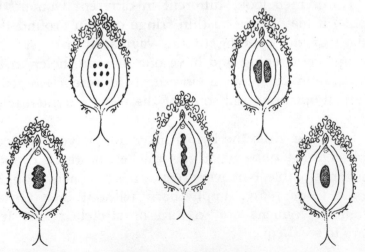

Illustration 26. Hymens

When the hymen is stretched or torn—whether it's during sex or while a girl's doing gymnastics or riding a horse or whatever—it may bleed a little, a whole lot, or not at all. It may hurt a little, a whole lot, or not at all. But only rarely does a hymen bleed or hurt so badly that a doctor's care is needed. In fact, most girls and women never notice any blood or feel any pain when their hymen is stretched or torn.

THE VAGINA, UTERUS, AND OVARIES

Another change that happens in a girl's body during puberty is that the sex organs on the inside of her body being to develop and grow. (Turn back to Illustration 6, page 38, to see these organs again.) The vagina gets longer, until it reaches its adult length of three to four inches. This still isn't very large, and as you may recall, the average penis is about six inches long when it's erect. But the vagina is very elastic and stretchy, so the penis can easily fit inside when a man and a woman are having sexual intercourse.

The uterus also gets larger during puberty, although even in a grown woman it is only about the size of a clenched fist. It, too, is very elastic and stretchy and can expand to accommodate a growing baby. Indeed, when a woman gives birth, both the uterus and vagina are stretched quite a bit.

The ovaries, the two egg-shaped organs on either side of the uterus, also grow larger during puberty. In grown women, they are about 1½ to 2 inches in size.

Just as a boy begins to make sperm in his testicles for the first time during puberty, so girls begin producing the first fully mature ova in their ovaries at this time. But unlike males, who are constantly making new sperm in their bodies, females have all the ova they'll ever have when they're born. They don't make new ova every day. The ova they have when they're born are not fully mature or ripe, however. The first ovum doesn't fully ripen and leave the ovary until after a girl has already started puberty and begun to develop pubic hair and breasts.

During puberty, a girl *ovulates* for the first time. A ripe ovum leaves her ovary; in fact, it pops right off. This process of popping a ripe ovum off the ovary is called *ovulation*. As soon as the ovum pops off, the fringed ends of the fallopian tubes reach out like tiny fingers to grasp the ovum and pull it into the tube. (see Illustration 27). The fallopian tubes are very tiny, no bigger around than a strand of spaghetti and only about four inches long. The inside of each tube is lined with tiny hairs, which are connected to the muscles in the walls of the tubes. The muscles contract and loosen up rhythmically. This causes the tiny hairs to sway back and forth and to sweep the ovum along the length of the tube toward the uterus.

If a girl has sexual intercourse at just about the time she releases her first ripe ovum, and if the boy has ejaculated sperm into her vagina, it's possible that one of his sperm could swim through her uterus, into her tubes, and meet up with and fertilize her first ripe ovum. But this doesn't usually happen. For one thing, most girls ovulate and produce their first ripe ovum when they're only about thirteen, and most girls of this age don't have sexual intercourse.

Even if a girl *did* have sexual intercourse just around the time that she released her first ovum from her ovary,

ovulates (AHV-u-lates)
ovulation (ahv-u-LAY-shun)

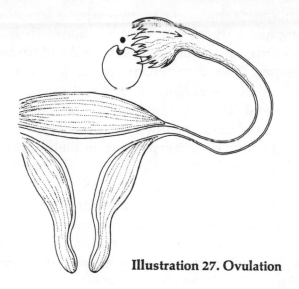

Illustration 27. Ovulation

and a sperm met up with it in the fallopian tube, the ovum probably wouldn't be fertilized by the sperm. The first ovum isn't really a fully mature one. It's sort of a "practice" ovum. It's *possible* for one of these "practice" ova to be fertilized, but it's very unusual. Usually, then, a girl's first ovum travels to the uterus without being fertilized. After a few days of floating around inside the uterus, the ovum simply disintegrates.

HORMONES

Like boys, girls begin to make new hormones in their bodies during puberty. As you may recall from reading Chapter 4, there's a gland in a boy's brain called the pituitary gland, and a few years before puberty it starts to make small amounts of certain hormones. These hormones travel to a boy's testicles and cause them to start making a hormone of their own called testosterone. At first, neither his pituitary nor his testicles make very much hormone, but as he grows older, a boy makes increasing amounts of pituitary hormones in his brain. This, in turn, causes his testicles to make more and more testosterone. The testosterone travels to other parts of his body and causes changes such as the enlargement of his penis and scrotum, the growth of pubic, facial, and body hair, and the lowering of his voice.

Girls, too, have pituitary glands in their brains. A few years before puberty begins, a girl's pituitary gland starts making the same hormones that a boy's pituitary makes. In girls, though, these pituitary hormones travel to the ovaries. Like the testicles, the ovaries are also glands and are also capable of making hormones. One of the hormones that a girl's ovaries make is called *estrogen*.

As she grows older, a girl's brain makes increasing amounts of pituitary hormone. This, in turn, causes her ovaries to make increasing amounts of estrogen. Just as testosterone from a boy's testicles travels to other parts of his body and causes puberty changes like pubic hair and the growth of his penis, so estrogen from a girl's ovaries travels to other parts of her body and causes certain puberty changes. For instance, estrogen is responsible for the growth of her pubic hair and the development of her breasts.

Estrogen also causes changes on the inside of a girl's uterus. The uterus is a hollow organ. The inside walls of the uterus are covered by a special lining. Before puberty, this lining is very thin. Once puberty starts and a girl is making increasing amounts of estrogen, this lining begins to grow thicker. It becomes very spongy and soft and fills with blood. By the time a girl has begun her growth spurt, sprouted pubic hair, and de-

estrogen (ES-tro-jen)

veloped breasts, the lining of her uterus has grown quite thick.

Like the other changes that happen during puberty, this takes place because a girl's body is getting ready for a time in her life when she may decide to have a baby. When and if she does become pregnant, this lining is very important. After her ovum is fertilized by a sperm in the fallopian tube, it will travel to the uterus and plant itself in the thick lining there. The lining will provide the blood and nutrients a fertilized ovum needs in order to grow into a baby.

THE MENSTRUAL PERIOD

As we've explained, a girl's first ovum isn't fertilized by a sperm. It doesn't plant itself in the uterine lining; instead, it simply disintegrates. Because the ovum hasn't been fertilized, there's no longer any need for the thick lining that has grown on the inside walls of the uterus, so the uterus begins to shed the lining. The tissues of the bloody lining begin to break up and turn very liquidy. The bloody and liquidy tissue collect at the bottom of the uterus. They dribble out the opening in the bottom of the uterus that leads to the vagina. Then the blood and liquid flow down the vaginal walls and dribble out the vaginal opening (see Illustration 28).

When a girl begins bleeding from her vaginal opening, we say she is *menstruating* or having her *menstrual period*. A girl generally has her first menstrual period sometime between the ages of nine and sixteen. The average age is about thirteen. It takes about three to seven days for the uterus to completely shed the lining.

menstruating (MEN-stroo-ate-ing)
menstrual (MEN-strool)

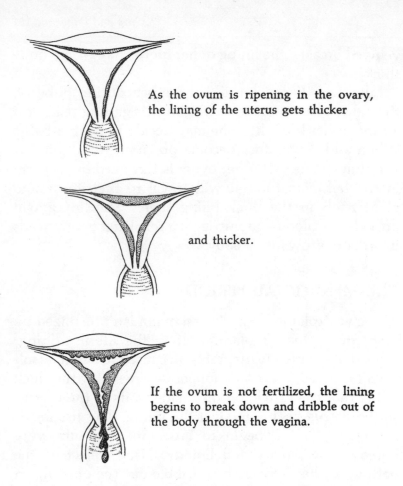

As the ovum is ripening in the ovary, the lining of the uterus gets thicker

and thicker.

If the ovum is not fertilized, the lining begins to break down and dribble out of the body through the vagina.

Illustration 28. Cross section of the uterus. The shaded area is the lining of the uterus. It breaks down and is shed during menstruation.

Altogether, about half a cup of blood comes out of the girl's vagina during her menstrual period. While she's bleeding like this, a girl usually wears a pad of cotton, called a sanitary pad or napkin, inside her underpants to catch the blood. Or she may insert a cotton plug, called a tampon, into her vagina to absorb the blood (see Illustration 29). She changes this pad or tampon several times a day.

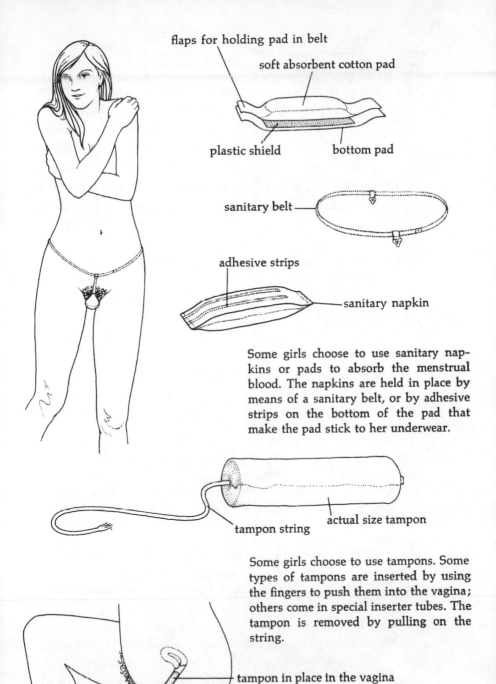

flaps for holding pad in belt

soft absorbent cotton pad

plastic shield　　　　bottom pad

sanitary belt

adhesive strips

sanitary napkin

Some girls choose to use sanitary napkins or pads to absorb the menstrual
blood. The napkins are held in place by
means of a sanitary belt, or by adhesive
strips on the bottom of the pad that
make the pad stick to her underwear.

actual size tampon

tampon string

Some girls choose to use tampons. Some
types of tampons are inserted by using
the fingers to push them into the vagina;
others come in special inserter tubes. The
tampon is removed by pulling on the
string.

tampon in place in the vagina

vaginal opening

Illustration 29. Sanitary napkins and tampon

The Menstrual Cycle

After the uterus has completely shed the lining and the girl stops bleeding, the lining starts to grow thick and spongy again. While this is happening, the ovaries are getting ready to ovulate again. About ten days or so after a girl finishes her menstrual bleeding, another ovum pops off one of her ovaries. It, too, travels through the fallopian tube toward the uterus. Unless it is fertilized by a sperm in the tube, it won't plant in the uterine lining either and will once again disintegrate.

Because the ovum hasn't been fertilized, the newly grown lining isn't needed. So it breaks down and dribbles out of the uterus into the vagina, and the process starts up again:

- The girl starts bleeding.
- The bleeding lasts for a few days or maybe a week or so, and then it stops.
- The lining of the uterus starts to grow thick and spongy again.
- The ovary releases another ripe ovum.
- The fingerlike ends of the fallopian tube grasp the ovum and pull it into the tube.
- The hairs inside the tube sweep the ovum toward the uterus.
- Unless the ovum is fertilized, it disintegrates inside the uterus.
- The newly grown lining breaks down and dribbles down the vaginal walls and out the vaginal opening.
- The girl starts bleeding and having another menstrual period.

The whole process, which is called the menstrual cycle, takes about a month. The cycle repeats itself, month after month, over and over again, year in and year out, throughout most of a woman's life. Once she gets to be about forty-five to fifty-five years old, the cycle stops. The woman stops ovulating and menstruating each month. This stopping of the monthly cycle is called *menopause*.

Between puberty, the time when she first starts menstruating, and menopause, the time when she stops menstruating, a female generally has her period pretty regularly, about once a month. This isn't a hard and fast rule, though. There are lots of exceptions. For one thing, women stop menstruating when they get pregnant. If a sperm fertilizes an ovum in the fallopian tube, the fertilized ovum travels to the uterus and plants itself in the uterine lining. The lining provides the blood and nourishment the fertilized ovum needs to grow into a baby. So for the nine months of her pregnancy, while the baby is growing inside her uterus, a woman doesn't shed her uterine lining. (Here again, there are exceptions to the rule; occasionally, a woman will have one or even two periods after she's gotten pregnant. But such periods are shorter than normal periods, and most women don't have their periods at all once the ovum has been fertilized.) After childbirth, the woman's periods may start up again within a few weeks or a month or two, or it may take several months before they start again.

Also, young girls who've just started menstruating don't always have their periods regularly, once a month. It usually takes a while for the body to adjust to menstruating. Many girls have their first period and then don't have a second one for a number of months. Some have their second period just a couple of weeks after their first. Girls often don't start having their periods very regularly until they've been menstruating for two or three years.

menopause (MEN-o-paws)

There are certain medical problems that can cause a woman to miss one or more menstrual periods or to stop menstruating altogether. Even healthy women without a single medical problem sometimes miss a period or two. Gaining or losing a lot of weight, moving to a new home, traveling, stress, excitement, nervousness, emotional ups and downs—all these things can cause a woman to miss her period. And there are some perfectly healthy women who only menstruate a few times a year. That's just the way their particular bodies work.

Most of the time, though, *most* women have their menstrual periods pretty regularly, about once a month. By "pretty regularly," we don't mean that it happens once every thirty days exactly. There's a lot of variation. Some women have periods that come as close together as every twenty-one days; others have periods that come as far apart as every thirty-six days. The average is about twenty-eight days.

No woman's period is like clockwork. One month the menstrual cycle may last twenty-five days; the next month it may last twenty-eight days; and the following month, thirty days. One month the bleeding may last for three days, the next month for five days. Some women's periods vary quite a bit, and others are more regular. In general, though, a woman's period comes about once a month and lasts for a few days to a week or so.

The First Period
Some girls are excited about the prospect of having their periods; others aren't so eager. Many girls are concerned that their first period will sneak up on them. They worry that the blood will soak through their

clothes without their realizing it and they'll be publicly embarrassed. Such things can happen, but generally a girl has a sensation of wetness and has plenty of time to get to the bathroom before the blood soaks through her underclothes. Besides, not that much blood comes out all at once. Altogether over the entire period, only about half a cup to a cup of blood is lost, so only a small amount is dribbling out of the vaginal opening at any one time.

Most girls use sanitary napkins or pads instead of tampons at first. A lot of girls think that a virgin, a girl who hasn't had sex yet, can't use a tampon because of the hymen. But as we explained, the hymen has openings in it and is very stretchy. Unless a girl has a particularly rigid or tight hymen, she can use a tampon regardless of whether or not she's had sexual intercourse. Still, most girls prefer to use napkins at first, unless they want to go swimming, in which case they use a tampon.

Menstrual Cramps
Menstrual cramps are abdominal pains that may occur early in the menstrual period or a few days before the period actually starts. Cramps may vary from a feeling of fullness or pressure, to a dull, achy feeling, to a sharp pain or spasm. Almost every woman has cramps at some time in her life, but for most they're not a real problem and don't interfere with their daily activities. There are, however, some women who have such severe cramps that they actually have to spend a few days in bed each month.

Severe cramps can be a sign of some underlying medical problem, and women who have severe cramps should see a doctor. Often, though, the doctor is unable to pinpoint a cause for the cramps. Many doctors used to think that cramps were "all in your head," and some doctors still think this. Recently, though, medical research has shown that women who have cramps often have unusually high levels of hormones called *prostaglandins*, which cause the uterus to contract painfully during menstruation. There are now anti-prostaglandin medications available to help such women. For most women, though, their cramps, if they have them at all, aren't uncomfortable enough for them to need medication. If they do need to take something, aspirin will usually do the trick.

Other Menstrual Changes

Some women notice other physical or emotional changes at certain points in their menstrual cycle. For example, I get very energetic during my period and often get into fits of housecleaning (which is nice because, most of the time, I'm not too enthusiastic about housework). About a week and a half before my period starts, my breasts swell a bit and get very tender, or sometimes downright painful. (This started happening only after I turned thirty.) For a couple of years after I turned thirty-two, I started having moderate cramps during the first couple of days of my period. I'd never had them before, and lately they seem to have disappeared again. I always know when I'm going to ovulate because I get to feeling very sexual.

Some girls and women don't notice any changes associated with their menstrual cycles; others do. Sometimes these changes are pleasant ones—extra energy, an especially "up" or good feeling, bursts of creativity. Sometimes they're negative—tension, irritability, head-

prostaglandins (pros-ta-GLAN-dins)

aches, bowel problems, swelling, and temporary weight gain. Some women notice that they're cranky right before their period starts, or that they are more apt to get depressed at this time. Some notice a slight twinge or cramps for a day or so about two weeks before their period starts. This is about when ovulation occurs, so this pain is sometimes called ovulation pain. For most women, though, the ovum pops off the ovary without their really noticing it.

Myths about Menstruation

People used to believe all sorts of crazy things about menstruation. Primitive tribes used to think that you'd get sick if you ate food cooked by a menstruating woman, that her glance could wither a field of crops, that having sex with a menstruating woman could make a man's penis fall off. Some tribes even banished women to menstrual huts each month during their period. Some of the slang terms used for menstruation—"the curse," "falling off the roof," "on the rag"—reflect these old, negative attitudes toward menstruation.

Today, we know that none of these things is true. A woman can have sex while she's menstruating and no harm will come to her sex partner. In fact, a menstruating woman can do anything during her period that she'd do at any other time. Old notions have a way of hanging on, though, and there are still some people who think that a menstruating woman shouldn't have sex, take a bath, wash her hair, drink cold drinks, or exercise, and that doing these things will cause a heavier flow, make her period last longer, or give her cramps. None of these things is true. In fact, sexual intercourse and exercise are often helpful for women who are troubled by cramps.

In the first six chapters of this book, we've tried to answer the questions you may have had about how puberty happens. But there may still be other questions you'd like answered. In Chapter 7 we will talk about a number of other topics related to puberty and sexuality, and you may find the answers to your questions there.

CHAPTER 7

Sexuality

Questions about sexuality come up all the time during puberty because, as we go through puberty, many of us experience stronger sexual feelings than ever before in our lives. For some, this means the urge to masturbate more often or to spend more time having sexual fantasies. For others, it means having very strong sexual and romantic attractions to someone or spending more time having fantasies in which they imagine a passionate romance with a special someone. These sexual and romantic feelings can be very intense and distracting. It may seem as if sex and romance are all you can think about. It helps to know that these feelings are perfectly normal and that a lot of other people your age are going through the same thing.

As they move through puberty and into the teen years, many boys start dating. Once a boy starts dating, he may find himself having to make decisions about sexuality. Is it all right to kiss on your first date? What about French-kissing (putting your tongue in

161

someone's mouth as you're kissing)? Is necking or making out (spending time kissing and hugging) okay? What about moving beyond making out and into petting "above the waist" (touching a girl's breasts) or "below the waist" (touching and rubbing the other person's genitals)? How about oral sex (using your mouth and tongue to stimulate the other person's sex organs)? What about sexual intercourse? When is it okay to have these kinds of sexual experiences and when is it not okay? In the following pages we'll be talking about this aspect of sexuality, and answering questions boys have about this topic.

We'll also be talking about other aspects of sexuality. People tend to think that sexuality refers just to having sexual intercourse, but it encompasses much more. Masturbation, kissing, touching yourself or someone else in a sexual way, being attracted to another person, having romantic or sexual feelings or fantasies—all these things are part of our sexuality. It would take an entire book (or maybe several books) to discuss sexuality thoroughly. So, in this chapter, we're just going to mention certain aspects of sexuality, concentrating on some of the problems and issues that may come up as you move through puberty and into your teen years. We'll also suggest other books in the section For Further Reading and other sources of information that might prove helpful.

SEX PLAY

People used to think that children didn't have sexual feelings or much interest in anything sexual until they reached puberty. We now know that children often have sexual feelings and are curious about sex at a very young age. Many children play sex games, such as "doctor," and this is a normal part of growing up. However, they often feel uncertain or uncomfortable about it. They ask questions like:

Is it wrong to "play doctor"? If two little kids fool around with each other, is it okay?
Although most adults don't approve of this kind of thing, the fact of the matter is that sex play is a normal part of learning about sex, and it doesn't mean that there's something wrong with you. However, bullying someone else or being bullied into sex play can be harmful. If you are bullied into doing something sexual by another child, or for that matter by anyone, it's important that you talk this problem over with your parents or another grown-up you trust.

If two guys fool around with each other, does this mean they're homosexual?
As we explained back in Chapter 5, homosexuality means having sexual thoughts, feelings, fantasies, or activities that involve someone who is the same sex as you are. But being a homosexual doesn't mean that a person *never* has any heterosexual feelings or activities. By the same token, being a heterosexual (having most of one's sexual feelings and activities involve people of the opposite sex) doesn't mean that a person never has homosexual feelings or actual experiences with a person of the same sex. In fact, almost one-third of the heterosexual men in this country have had at least one homosexual experience with another man to the point of orgasm at some point in their lives. We'll talk more about homosexuality in the next section, but for now you should know that "fooling around," which may include such things as kissing, hugging, masturbating, and/or oral-genital sex, with another boy does not mean that a boy is a homosexual.

HOMOSEXUALITY

Although most adults in our society are heterosexuals, about one in ten are homosexuals. "Gay" is another term for homosexuals, and female homosexuals are also called lesbians.

People get the idea that people are either strictly homosexual or strictly heterosexual, but, as we explained above, this isn't true. To be strictly heterosexual, *all* of a person's thoughts, feelings, fantasies, and actual sexual experiences throughout his or her whole life would have to center around people of the opposite sex. To be strictly homosexual, all of a person's thoughts, feelings, fantasies, and sexual experiences throughout his or her entire life would only be about people of the same sex. Very, very few people are strictly heterosexual or strictly homosexual. Most of us, regardless of whether we're mostly homosexual or mostly heterosexual, have at least some feelings in the other direction at some time in our life. But when we use the term *homosexual*, we're talking about people whose strongest sexual feelings are for people of the same sex. The term *bisexual* is used to describe people whose sexual attractions and activities are about equally divided between the two sexes.

Is homosexuality wrong?
Different people have different ideas about what is morally wrong or sinful. Some people consider homosexuality morally wrong or sinful; others don't. Some people view homosexuality as a mental sickness and feel that homosexuals need psychological help to "cure" them. Still others don't feel that homosexu-

lesbians (LEZ-be-anz)

ality is either wrong or a sign of sickness. They feel that some people just happen to be homosexuals, that it's a personal matter, and that there's nothing wrong or sick about it.

Why are some people homosexuals?
Although people have various theories about this, the truth of the matter is that no one knows the answer to this question.

MAKING DECISIONS ABOUT SEX

The kids in my classes have a *lot* of questions about this topic. Many times, the way they ask these questions tells me that they have the idea in the back of their heads that there is some definite set of rules you're supposed to follow or certain steps you're supposed to take as far as sex is concerned. They ask things like:

How old should a person be before he or she has sex? How do you know if you're ready for sex? Should you wait till you're married?
Even though each of these questions is phrased a bit differently, they are all about the same thing—when is it okay to have sex, and when isn't it okay? If there were a set of rules that everyone agreed to, these would be easy questions to answer. But there aren't any agreed-upon rules, and different people have different ideas on this subject.

In class, at least in the classes for older kids, we spend a lot of time on these questions. We don't usually come up with clear answers that work for everyone, but we at least discuss the issue, and I try to present the various different ideas that different people have and to explain why they have these ideas.

Some people have what I call "the legal point of

view." In most states, there are laws that make it illegal (against the law) for people under a certain age to have sex. These laws vary from state to state. In some states, it's as young as fourteen; in others, it's sixteen, eighteen, or twenty-one. These laws are rarely enforced, but they are laws. People who take the legal point of view feel that you shouldn't have sex until you've reached whatever the legal age is in your state. But very few people who have definite ideas about when a person should start to have sex are actually concerned about law. In fact, for many people, it's not *how old* you are that is the important thing. Many people feel that you shouldn't have sex until you're married, regardless of your age.

People who have the "wait until you're married" point of view may have this opinion for a variety of different reasons. For some, it's a religious thing. They feel that the Bible tells us very clearly that people should not have sex unless they're married to each other. For others, it has more to do with pregnancy. Such people are concerned about what will happen if an unmarried couple have sex and the woman (or girl) gets pregnant. They point out that even if a couple uses birth control, it's still possible for the woman to get pregnant. They feel that a decision to have sex isn't just a decision between two people but a choice that involves the responsibility for a possible third person, the baby that might be conceived. For this reason, they feel that you shouldn't have sex until you're married, engaged to be married, and/or ready to take on the responsibility of raising a child.

There are also other reasons why people have the "wait until you're married" point of view. One man we interviewed (who was not a religious man) explained this point of view particularly well:

My wife and I waited until we were married to have sex, which was a different decision than many people nowadays make. But I think it was a good one. Maybe if we'd had sex with other people or with each other before we were married, we'd have been more experienced or knowledgeable. But learning about sex together, with each other, made it that much more special. Also, we didn't have to worry if either of us was "as good" as the other lovers either of us might have had before, so we didn't have the jealous, uncertain feelings some couples have.

By being willing to wait until we were married, I felt I was showing her that it wasn't just sex that I wanted from her but real, true love and lifelong commitment with her. And she was showing me the same thing, that we really mattered to each other as people, beyond just a physical, sexual wanting or desire. We really trusted each other, and that made us feel safe enough for us to really "let go." We didn't have to worry that if we did it "wrong" or it wasn't great the first time that it would all be over. And, really, it wasn't so great the first time. It was kind of awkward and embarrassing. But I knew and she knew that we'd both be around tomorrow. So we were able to be free and open and to make mistakes and to learn how to make love. If we hadn't been married and hadn't already promised to be there through thick and thin with each other, I think it would have been harder to learn to have good sex. We might have had hurt feelings or uncertainties or shynesses that we couldn't have gotten past. But by the fact of marrying, we had already promised ourselves to "work things out, come what may." This trusting and promising made us able to grow to be better lovers than we might have otherwise.

Charlie, age 67

People who have the "legal" point of view, people like Charlie, and other people who have the "wait until you're married" point of view have very clear-cut answers to the questions about when it's okay and when it's not okay to have sex. But for many people, these answers aren't so clear-cut. Some people feel it's okay for two people to have sexual intercourse as long as they're both adults, which for some people means a specific age, such as eighteen or twenty-one. For some people, it's not so much a specific age but that both people are mature enough to "handle it." Others feel that people shouldn't have sex unless they're "really in love" or are committed to a long-term relationship. The problem with this is, How do you know if you're mature enough to "handle it," if you're "really in love," or if the other person is really in love with you? There aren't any easy answers to these questions.

People who feel that two people shouldn't have sex until they're mature enough to handle it or unless they're really in love are concerned about the emotional feelings involved in sex. Having sexual intercourse involves our deepest emotional feelings, and it's very easy for people to be hurt. When parents don't want teenagers to have sex, many times they're concerned not only about the possibility of pregnancy but also about the possibility of the emotional pain that can happen when two people have sex and the relationship then ends, with one person or both having to suffer emotionally. Also, as Charlie pointed out, sex is something that takes some time to work out. If two people aren't in love or in a long-term relationship that guarantees that the other person will be around to work things out with, one or both people may suffer emotionally.

Making a decision about sex isn't always an easy thing to do. There's often a great deal of pressure on teenagers to have sex, and many young people are pressured into having sex before they're really ready to do so. If you've wondered about how you'd know whether or not you're ready to have sex, it helps to talk the issue over with someone—your parents, other adults you trust, and friends. Also, you might find *Changing Bod-*

ies, Changing Lines, one of the books listed in For Further Reading at the end of this book, particularly helpful. It has an excellent section on teens and sexual decision making.

What's the first thing you should do when you have sex?
Could you explain to us, step by step, what people do
when they're having sex?
As we've said, sexual intercourse isn't something that has specific rules you have to follow. When kids go out to the playground after school, they don't have a specific set of directions. No one tells them that first they must take five steps, then do three somersaults, then swing on the swing for five minutes, then climb to the top of the jungle gym. They just go out there and fool around and play and do whatever they feel like doing.

When I say this to the kids in my classes, I don't mean to suggest that having sexual intercourse is like going out to the playground to fool around (although there is a certain playfulness that can happen when two people are having sex). The point I'm trying to make is that there just aren't any rules or instructions, or a "right way" to have sexual intercourse.

Some people like to hug and kiss a lot first. Some like to French-kiss (put their tongues into the other person's mouth while kissing); others don't like this much. Touching, kissing, and hugging usually give people warm, excited, sexual feelings. The couple may then touch each other's genitals before intercourse, which is called foreplay; they may also engage in oral-genital sex (using their mouths to stimulate each other's genital organs).

When questions about oral-genital sex come up in the question box, many kids go, "Oh, yuck, why would anyone want to do that?" I explain that many couples find this a very pleasurable way of enjoying each other's bodies and a special way of being close. It's also a way of being sexual with someone that doesn't involve the possibility of the woman's getting pregnant. I think many kids find the idea of oral-genital sex kind of gross because they think of this area of the body as being "dirty" or full of germs. Actually, though, this area of our bodies isn't any dirtier or more germ-laden than other parts of our bodies. In fact, most people's mouths have more germs than their genitals.

Another thing that bothers kids when they hear about something like oral-genital sex is that they think that it's something you *have* to do when you have sex. This isn't true. Some couples enjoy oral-genital sex and often include it in their lovemaking. Others don't feel comfortable with it and rarely, if ever, do it. When you grow up, you may decide that it's something you'd like to try, or you may decide it's not something you ever want to try. It's normal if you do and normal if you don't. Like everything else about sex, you're the one who gets to decide.

PREGNANCY

Whenever we discuss sexuality and sexual intercourse, questions about pregnancy and childbirth naturally come up. It would take another whole book to explain everything about pregnancy. But we'll try to answer at least the most common questions that come up in our classes.

Are there only certain times of the month when a girl can get pregnant? If so, when?
A woman's ovum can be fertilized only during the thirty-six hours (some experts say forty-eight hours)

right after she's ovulated. It's only in this first day or so after the ovum has popped off the ovary that the ovum is at the exact ripeness to allow for fertilization. After that, the egg is "overripe" and cannot be fertilized. Within a few days, it will break down and disintegrate completely.

Because there's only, at most, forty-eight hours in which a woman's ovum can be fertilized during each menstrual cycle, it would seem to be a pretty easy thing to avoid getting pregnant: just don't have sex during those forty-eight hours. Unfortunately, it's not that simple. First of all, sperm can stay alive in the woman's body for up to three (some experts say five) days. So let's say a woman ovulated on the tenth of the month. If she'd had sex on the seventh and the man had ejaculated, the sperm could still be in her body, alive and well, waiting for the ovum when it popped off the ovary on the tenth.

Also, there's no way to predict ahead of time exactly when a woman is going to ovulate. A woman usually ovulates twelve to sixteen days before the first day of bleeding of her menstrual period. So we can count backward and get an idea of when she ovulated in the *previous* cycle, but we can't tell when she'll ovulate in the *next* cycle. As we explained in Chapter 6, women's menstrual cycles aren't always regular. One month, a woman's cycle may last twenty-eight days, the next month thirty-two, and the next twenty-one. Even women who have fairly regular periods—say, every twenty-seven or twenty-eight days—will occasionally have longer or shorter than usual periods. There's just no way of telling ahead of time exactly when a woman will ovulate.

I heard that if you only have sex during your period,
you won't get pregnant. Is this true?

No; it *is* possible for a woman to get pregnant if she has
sex while she's menstruating, that is, while she's having her menstrual period. A woman whose period lasts
for longer than the usual seven days is more likely to
get pregnant from having sex during her period. But
even a woman whose period lasts seven days or less
could get pregnant from having sex during this time.

Here's an example of how this might work. Say Mary
starts her period on June 3. She bleeds for seven days,
until June 9. She has sex on June 8, while she's still
bleeding. Her next period starts on June 24. Altogether,
twenty-one days have elapsed between the first day of
bleeding of her period on June 3 and the first day of
bleeding of her next period on June 24. By counting
back twelve to sixteen days from June 24, we can figure
that she probably ovulated between the twelfth and
eighth of June. Mary was still bleeding on the eighth;
she may have ovulated on the eighth; she had sex on the
eighth. There's a good chance she'd get pregnant even
though she was having her period.

Even if she didn't ovulate until the ninth or tenth, she
still might get pregnant because the sperm can stay
alive for three days. And if the experts who say sperm
can stay alive for *five* days are right, she might have
gotten pregnant from having sex on the eighth even if
she didn't ovulate until the twelfth.

Or, to take another example, let's say Susan has a
period on August 1. She bleeds for seven days, until
August 7. She has sex on the seventh day, that's August
7, while she's still bleeding. Her next period starts on
August 28, which would mean she'd had a twenty-
seven-day cycle. So she may have ovulated as early as
August 12. She stopped bleeding on the seventh. But

if the experts who say that sperm can stay alive for five days are right, there might still be some live sperm in her body from the time she had sex on August 7. Therefore, when she ovulated on August 12, she could become pregnant from having had sex on the seventh while she was still bleeding.

It is, then, possible for a woman to get pregnant from having sex during her menstrual period.

How old does a girl have to be before she can get pregnant?
Could a girl get pregnant before she's even had her first period?
Once a girl reaches puberty and begins to menstruate and ovulate, she is physically capable of becoming pregnant. As we explained in Chapter 6 (see pages 148–149), it is possible for a girl to get pregnant before she's had her first period, but it isn't very likely.

Can a girl get pregnant the first time she has sex?
A lot of kids think that a girl can't get pregnant the first time she has sex. *This is not true.* Once a girl has begun to ovulate, to produce a ripe ovum each month or so, she can get pregnant, even if she's only had sex one time.

Does a girl have to have sex to get pregnant?
If a sperm meets up with an ovum and fertilizes it, the girl (or woman) can become pregnant. The most common way that a sperm and an ovum meet up is when a man and a woman have sexual intercourse around the time that she ovulates and the man ejaculates sperm into the woman's vagina. If the man only ejaculated sperm *near* the opening of the vagina, it is still possible for the sperm to swim into the vagina, up into the uterus, and to the fallopian tube, where it could fertilize the ovum. Even if a man were to pull his penis out of

the vagina and ejaculate in such a way that none of the sperm got into the vagina or near the vaginal opening, the woman might still get pregnant. As a man gets sexually aroused and his penis gets erect, a couple of drops of fluid may appear at the tip of his penis. This fluid may contain a few sperm, and most experts think that just these few sperm could cause pregnancy.

There are also special medical procedures doctors use to help women who are having problems getting pregnant.

These are the *only* ways in which a female can become pregnant. A girl or woman can't get pregnant from kissing, masturbating, sitting on a guy's lap, sitting on a toilet seat, or, indeed, any other ways except the ones we've mentioned.

How old is a woman before she's too old to have a baby?
As we explained in Chapter 6, women stop having babies when they've gone through menopause. Menopause is a time in a woman's life when her ovaries stop producing a ripe ovum each month and she stops having her menstrual periods. Menopause usually happens between the ages of forty-five and fifty-five, although it does happen earlier or later than this for some women.

As far as I know, the oldest woman who ever had a baby was a fifty-six-year-old grandmother from Glendale, California. Although her periods were coming only once in a while, the woman had not yet gone through menopause. She had sexual intercourse, and much to her surprise, she got pregnant. She gave birth to a normal, healthy baby.

Why are some babies girls and some boys?
The sex of the baby depends on the father's sperm. Some sperm have what scientists call an "x factor,"

which means they are capable of uniting with an ovum and making a female baby. Other sperm have a "y factor," which means they are capable of uniting with an ovum and making a male baby. If a y-factor sperm fertilizes the ovum, the baby will be a boy. If an x-factor sperm fertilizes the ovum, the baby will be a girl.

Could a girl have a penis? Can a person be both sexes at once?
Normally, a girl couldn't have a penis, and people are either one sex or the other. However, there are a few people called *hermaphrodites*, who have both male and female sex organs. Hermaphrodites generally have both testicles and ovaries on the inside of their bodies. On the outside, they may look a number of different ways. A hermaphrodite might, for example, have a penis and a man's body build, but have breasts like a woman. A hermaphrodite can also look like a woman, with a curvy body shape, breasts, and no beard, yet have a penis instead of the female genital organs. Or a hermaphrodite might have a vulva with inner and outer lips and a penis instead of a clitoris.

When I explain to my class about hermaphrodites, I usually see a few kids gulping and looking very nervous and worried. The girls who are late starters and haven't gotten their menstrual periods or whose breasts haven't started to develop start wondering if they really are females. If they've started to grow a few dark hairs on their upper lips—which sometimes happens to girls during puberty—they're apt to worry, "Oh no, maybe I'm growing a mustache and am really a hermaphrodite." Some of the boys look worried, too, especially if they've noticed the kind of breast swelling we talked about in

hermaphrodites (her-MAF-row-dites)

Chapter 4. They think maybe they're growing breasts and aren't really boys at all.

I tell them to relax. For one thing, hermaphroditism is very rare. Besides, hermaphrodites are generally mentally retarded, so if you're smart enough to go to school and be reading this book, you don't need to worry about being a hermaphrodite.

How do twins happen? How come twins don't always look alike? If a woman has twins, do they both come out at the same time?
Twins can happen in one of two ways: either there are two fertilized seeds, or there is one fertilized seed that splits into two (see Illustration 30).

Usually, a woman's ovaries produce only one ripe ovum a month. Occasionally, though, a woman will produce two ripe ova at the same time. If both of these ova are fertilized and plant themselves in the lining of the uterus, the woman will have twins. Twins that grow from two separate ova, fertilized by two separate sperm, are called *fraternal twins*. One may be a boy and one a girl, or they may both be the same sex. They won't necessarily look alike.

The other type of twins are called *identical twins*. Identical twins happen when the fertilized ovum and sperm split into two shortly after fertilization. No one knows why this happens. Twins that come from the same ovum and sperm look almost exactly alike and are always the same sex.

When twins are born, one comes out first and the other comes out within a few minutes. In some cases, it takes more than a few minutes for the second twin to be born; there have even been times when it took a whole day. But usually, twins are born within a few minutes of each other.

fraternal (freh-TUR-nul)

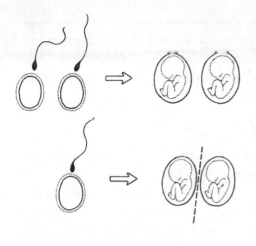

Sometimes a woman will produce two ripe ova the same month. If each of these ova is fertilized by sperm, the woman will have fraternal twins.

At other times, a sperm may fertilize a single ripe ovum. Then, after fertilization, the ovum splits into two, and the woman will have identical twins.

Illustration 30. Twins

What about triplets? What are the most babies a woman ever had at one time?

Triplets (three babies), quadruplets (four), quintuplets (five), sextuplets (six), septuplets (seven), and octuplets (eight), happen less frequently than twins.

Once you start getting more than three babies at a time, the chances of all the babies surviving is lower. Because there are so many of them, they're smaller than normal babies, and they're usually born prematurely; that is, before they've had a chance to fully develop. I think the largest number of babies born at one time is twelve, but not all of them survived. I think the largest number that ever lived was eight, or possibly nine.

I'm not sure of the exact numbers because the numbers are always changing. Nowadays, doctors have drugs, called fertility drugs, that they give to women who haven't been able to get pregnant because they don't ovulate. These drugs "jazz up" the ovary and cause the woman to ovulate. The problem is that they jazz up the ovaries so much that the woman produces not one but several ripe ova at a time. Newer and stronger drugs are constantly being developed. As a result, the number of babies born to a woman at any one time is always increasing.

What are Siamese twins?
Siamese twins are identical twins who are born with their bodies attached to each other in some way. Siamese twins happen when the fertilized ovum is splitting into two, making identical twins. For some unknown reason, the split is not completed and the babies develop so that some parts of their bodies are joined together.

Identical twins are pretty rare. Siamese twins are even rarer. When Siamese twins do happen, they may be joined in a number of ways. For instance, they may be joined at the feet, the shoulders, or the arms. When they are attached in such places, they are generally fairly easy to separate. A doctor can operate (usually shortly after the babies are born) and cut the babies apart. But sometimes it's not so easy. The babies may be joined at the head or chest or in such a way that cutting them apart would kill one or both of them. The parents may decide to have the operation done even though one baby will die. If the parents decide not to have the operation, or if it's not possible to operate without killing both babies, the twins spend their lives attached to each other (Illustration 31).

BIRTH CONTROL

Birth control is another topic that often comes up when we talk about sexuality. If a couple want to have sexual intercourse, but don't want a pregnancy, they need to use some form of birth control. Other terms for birth

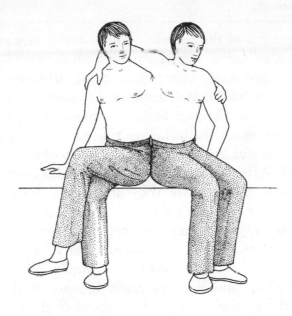

Illustration 31. Siamese twins

control include *contraception, contraceptives,* or *family planning.*

There are a number of different methods of birth control. One method, known as sterilization, involves an operation performed by a doctor. Males are sterilized by means of an operation called a *vasectomy,* in which the doctor uses a special drug to numb the scrotum and then cuts into the scrotum and severs each vas deferens (the tubes through which sperm travel out of the testicles). It is a simple operation that can be done in a doctor's office. Afterward, the man's testicles still make sperm, and he still has erections and ejaculates. But because each vas deferens has been cut, the sperm

contraception (kon-tre-SEP-shun)
contraceptives (kon-tre-SEP-tives)
sterilization (stare-a-lie-ZAY-shun)
vasectomy (vas-EK-te-me)

can't get out of the testicles. There aren't any sperm in the man's "come" when he ejaculates, so the woman can't get pregnant. The sperm simply disintegrate and disappear while in the testicles. Females are sterilized by an operation known as a *tubal ligation* or "tying the tubes," in which the fallopian tubes, the tubes through which the ova travel on their way to the uterus, are severed. Afterward, the woman's ovaries continue to make ova. But because the tubes have been cut, the sperm and ovum can't meet up with and fertilize each other, so no pregnancy can occur. (Again, the ovum simply disintegrates.) The woman's sterilization operation is a bit more involved than a man's. She has to be put to sleep and the operation has to be done in a hospital, but she's usually in and out of the hospital in less than one day.

There have been some cases in which the doctor has been able to resew the vas or the tubes after a man or woman has been sterilized so that pregnancy can occur. But most of the time, once people have been sterilized, they can't get pregnant or cause someone else to get pregnant ever again. Sterilization, then, is considered a permanent method of birth control and is usually used only by people who already have children and are quite sure they don't want any more.

There are also other, non-permanent methods that work as long as the couple use the method; once they stop using it, pregnancy can occur. Some of these methods, like the Pill, the IUD, and the diaphragm, require a doctor's prescription. The Pill, also known as an oral contraceptive, contains female hormones that prevent a woman from ovulating. The woman takes

ligation (lie-GAY-shun)
diaphragm (DIE-eh-fram)

one pill each day for three weeks and then takes a "week off," during which time she has her period. As long as she continues taking the pills on the three weeks on/one week off schedule, she is usually protected from getting pregnant, even if she has sex on the "off" week. Once she stops taking the pills altogether, or misses more than one pill a month, she is again susceptible to pregnancy.

The IUD, or intrauterine device, is a small piece of plastic inserted by a doctor or other trained medical person into the woman's uterus. Although no one is certain how or why it works, as long as the device remains in the uterus, the woman is usually protected from pregnancy. If she wishes to become pregnant, she must go back to the doctor and have the IUD removed. She can't remove it herself.

The diaphragm is a rubber, cuplike device that fits into the top of the woman's vagina. It is used with special sperm-killing chemicals called *spermicides* that are placed in the cup of the diaphragm. The woman puts the spermicide into the cup and places the diaphragm in her vagina before intercourse (as many as six hours before). She must leave it in place for at least eight hours after she has had sex to make sure all the sperm are dead. If she wants to have sex again during those eight hours, she does not remove the diaphragm. Instead, she uses a special applicator to insert more spermicide into her vagina. In order to work properly, the diaphragm has to be fitted for the first time by a doctor or nurse or other trained medical person.

In addition to the methods that require a doctor's prescription, there are also contraceptives that you can

intrauterine (in-tra-UTE-er-in)
spermicides (SPURM-eh-sides)

buy in a drugstore, pharmacy, or sometimes in a grocery store. Condoms or prophylactics—which are also known as "rubbers," "Trojans," and "safes"—are a male method of birth control. The condom is a rubber sheath that is placed over the erect penis just prior to intercourse. When the man ejaculates, the sperm are trapped in the condom, so they can't get into the woman's body.

Foam is another contraceptive that can be purchased without a doctor's prescription. It is a spermicide that comes in a pressurized container with a special applicator. Shortly before intercourse, the woman inserts an applicator full of foam into her vagina. When the man ejaculates, the sperm are killed by the spermicide in the foam. There are other spermicides that come in the form of creams or jellies and that are placed into the vagina by means of a special applicator shortly before intercourse. There are also spermicides that come in tablet form. These, too, are placed in the vagina before intercourse, and they melt and release their spermicides to kill the sperm ejaculated by the man. These sorts of spermicides are not, however, quite as effective as foam. Recently, a new method of birth control that can be purchased without a doctor's prescription has come on the market. Known as "the sponge," "the contraceptive sponge," or "the Today contraceptive sponge," this method involves a small, white, spongy device with a spermicide in it. It is soaked in water and placed into the top of the vagina before intercourse. Like a diaphram, it blocks the sperm from getting into the uterus, and the spermicide also works to kill the sperm.

Another method of birth control, called natural family planning, doesn't require a doctor's prescription or

prophylactics (pro-fe-LACK-tics)

buying any special creams or devices. It works by teaching a couple to recognize when a woman is about to ovulate, so the couple can avoid having intercourse at this time when the woman is apt to get pregnant. It involves keeping a calendar of the woman's menstrual cycles, taking her temperature every day (a woman's body temperature rises slightly around ovulation), and learning to recognize other body signs that let a woman know when ovulation is about to occur.

All these methods of birth control—sterilization, the Pill, the IUD, the diaphragm, the condom, foam, spermicides, the sponge, and natural family planning—are contraceptives. They prevent the ovum from being fertilized and/or planting itself in the uterine lining. However, even if the woman does get pregnant (because one of these methods was used but didn't work, because the method wasn't used properly, or because no method was used), there are still methods of birth control that prevent a woman from having a baby. In certain cases, the "morning-after pill," a hormone pill that is taken by a woman who fears that her ovum may have been fertilized, will prevent the fertilized ovum from planting in the lining of the uterus. But in order to work, the morning-after pill must be taken within at least three days of the time the woman had sexual intercourse. Another alternative would be for a woman to have an IUD inserted within a few days of having had intercourse. This will also prevent the fertilized ovum from planting itself in the uterus.

An abortion can be done if birth control has been ineffective or has not been used, and the woman has gotten pregnant and does not wish to have a baby. Abortions are done by doctors or other trained medical people; they remove the fertilized ovum and the lining from the pregnant woman's uterus. Most abortions are done in the first twelve weeks of preganancy, when the embryo (the fertilized ovum) is still very small and not very human or babylike. However, it is legal to do abortions up to twenty-six weeks of pregnancy.

As you may know, abortion is a very controversial topic. Some people think that abortion should be outlawed. They feel it is the same as murder. Other people feel that a woman should have the right to decide whether or not she wants to have a baby and that abortion is an individual decision between a woman and her doctor. They feel that the government doesn't have the right to make laws regulating what should or shouldn't go on inside a person's body.

When the topics of abortion and the various methods of birth control come up in class, kids have dozens and dozens of questions. They often want to know exactly how these various methods work to prevent pregnancy or how you go about using them. These questions are beyond the scope of this book. Luckily, there are some good books that do answer these questions that are listed in the For Further Reading section at the end of this book. Here, though, we'd like to answer some of the more general questions about birth control that kids ask.

Which methods work best?
No method is 100 percent effective. For example, a condom could break, the tubes could grow back together after a sterilization operation, or the Pill could fail to prevent a woman from producing a ripe ovum. However, when pregnancy occurs despite the fact that the couple used birth control, it's not usually the method that has failed; it's the user of the method who's at fault. For instance, a woman may forget to take her

pills, or she might neglect to put spermicide in her diaphragm.

What if the guy pulled his penis out so that
he didn't come inside the girl?
This is called the withdrawal method of birth control, and it doesn't work very well; in fact, it fails more than 80 percent of the time. It doesn't work because too often the man isn't able to control his ejaculation and doesn't withdraw in time. Also, there may be some sperm in the drop or so of lubrication that appears at the tip of the penis when it becomes erect, and these sperm could cause a pregnancy.

I heard that if you jump up and down after sex, you won't get
pregnant—true? Suppose a girl douches right after sex,
will this keep her from getting pregnant?
These questions refer to some of the common myths about preventing pregnancy. Jumping up and down after sex won't prevent pregnancy. Douching (washing the vagina out by means of a special douche bag or bottle) won't help either. Some people think that you can use plastic wrap such as Saran Wrap instead of a condom, but this won't prevent pregnancy because the sperm can leak out too easily. And, despite what you might have heard, a girl can get pregnant regardless of whether or not she has an orgasm.

Where could a teenager get birth control? Is it legal
for teenagers to have birth control?
The contraceptives that can be purchased in the drugstore or grocery store can be sold to anyone, regardless of age. Doctors are also allowed to prescribe birth control to anyone, regardless of age, and they are not re-

douches (DOO-shez)

quired to tell the parents if the person is under age. Many people, even if they are going to use one of the methods that doesn't require a doctor's prescription, choose to get their birth control method from a family planning clinic such as Planned Parenthood, because these clinics often have special classes to teach teens about birth control. Planned Parenthood clinics are usually listed in the white pages of the phone book or under "family planning clinics" in the yellow pages.

VENEREAL DISEASES AND OTHER HEALTH PROBLEMS

Venereal diseases, or VD, are infections that are usually passed from one person to another by some type of close sexual contact, such as sexual intercourse or oral-genital sex. Other terms for VD include sexually transmitted diseases (STDs), and sexually transmissible infections (STIs). In addition to VD, there are other health problems that can affect a man's genitals. In this section, we'll try to answer the most common questions about VD and other health problems.

Is VD just one disease or a whole bunch of different diseases? What kinds of VD are there?
There are actually a number of different kinds of VD. One thing that they all have in common is that they are caused by organisms that live in the soft mucous membranes of the human body; that is, in places like the mouth, the sex organs, and the rectum (the bowels). Another is that they are usually passed through sexual contact. They also tend to cause similar kinds of symptoms, which may include any of the following: unusual

venereal (ve-NEAR-e-ul)
mucous (MEW-cuss)

discharges from the penis or the vagina; burning or pain during urination; redness, pain, or itching of the sex organs; and sores, lumps, bumps, or blisters on the sex organs.

Although there are many different kinds of venereal diseases, people are usually thinking of either *gonorrhea, syphilis,* or *herpes* when they use the term *VD.*

How can a person get VD?
Generally speaking, VD is only passed by sexual contact. It is, however, possible for an infected woman to pass syphilis to her unborn child during pregnancy. Syphilis, gonorrhea, and herpes can also be passed to the baby during childbirth if the mother's vagina is infected. If a person who had a herpes or syphilis sore on his or her lip kissed someone, or touched a sore and immediately touched someone's genitals, anus, or mouth, he or she might pass the germs on.

Also, if you used a washcloth, drinking glass, or some other object that had been used by someone with herpes or syphilis *immediately* after that person had used it, it might be possible to get the germs. The germs that cause VD can live for only a few seconds outside the human body, though, and so they can't be passed from one person to another by objects like toilet seats. Most of the time, people get these infections through sexual contact.

Can VD be cured?
Yes. Most forms of VD can be cured if they're treated right away. If gonorrhea doesn't get treated until it's spread up into the uterus and tubes, it's possible for a

gonorrhea (gon-or-REE-a)
syphilis (SIF-ill-iss)
herpes (HER-peas)

woman to die from it or to be unable to have a baby after the infection is cured because it's left so much scar tissue. If syphilis gets to the point where it has caused blindness or insanity or other advanced symptoms, it may not be possible to cure it. Fortunately, the vast majority of cases of gonorrhea and syphilis are cured before they get this far.

Herpes can't be cured at present, at least not in the sense that there's a medicine that will get rid of the organisms in your body. But that doesn't mean the sores will always be there. Some people have one outbreak of sores, then the sores go away, and the germs retreat into the body, where they don't cause any problems and can't be passed on to someone else. But the germs are still there in the body, and, for most people, they will act up from time to time, causing new outbreaks of sores and making the person again become infectious (able to pass the infection on to someone else) for a period of time preceding, during, and following the outbreak of the sores.

How does a person know if he or she has got VD?
Usually, people know they've got VD because they develop symptoms and go to the doctor, who performs certain tests to find out what type of VD they have. However, in many cases, people with syphilis or gonorrhea don't notice the first symptoms. In women with gonorrhea, this can cause problems, because they may not know they have the disease until it has spread up into the uterus and tubes, where it can cause serious problems.

Because the early symptoms may go unnoticed, it's important for people who have VD to alert everyone they've had sex with recently to the fact that they have VD.

Where can you go to get treatment?
Your doctor can treat you. Public health departments will also test and treat you for free. For more information about treatment or any other questions about VD, see the books listed in For Further Reading (pages 208–211) or call the National VD Hotline. In California, call 1-800-982-5883; in other states, call 1-800-227-8922. The call is free and won't appear on your phone bill, and you don't have to give your name.

I've never had sex, but I have symptoms like you said you get
from VD. I have pain, and it burns when I urinate, and
sometimes a little bit of stuff leaks out of my penis.
If it's not VD, what is it?
There are a number of diseases other than VD that can cause these kinds of symptoms. Urethritis, an infection of the urethra, can cause pain in the genitals, a discharge, and pain or burning on urination. Sometimes urethritis is caused by germs that are passed through sexual contact, but you can also pick up germs that cause urethritis in other ways.

What are crabs, and how do you get them?
"Crabs," or pubic lice, are tiny, tiny bugs that attach themselves to pubic hair by means of their crablike claws and feed on the blood vessels under the skin. They cause intense itching. They can be passed during sexual contact, and it's also possible to pick them up from clothing, bed linen, mattresses, or anything that has been infested with the crabs or the tiny eggs they lay. They can be killed with special lice medicine such as Rid, which can be purchased without a prescription, or the doctor can prescribe a lotion called Kwell.

urethritis (YOUR-eh-THRI-tis)

What is jock itch?
"Jock itch" or "jock rot" is a fungus caused by wearing clothes that are too tight or that don't let the air circulate freely. This causes redness, soreness, and itching on the genitals and the inside of the thighs. Rubbing cornstarch on the area may be enough to cure the problem, but in some cases you need to get special medication from the doctor to clear it up. Keeping the area clean and dry, washing your clothes frequently, and avoiding tight clothing will help avoid the problem.

What would happen if a boy only had one testicle?
Most males are born with two testicles. Every once in a great while, someone is born with only one. Or a man or boy could have some sort of injury or accident that could crush one testicle so badly that it had to be removed.

If for one reason or another a man has only one testicle, the testicle he does have takes over for the missing testicle, and it will produce enough sperm so that he'll still be able to make a woman pregnant. His sex life and everything else about him will be completely normal.

What is an undescended testicle?
Before a boy is born, his testicles are up inside his body. Once he is born, they descend (come down) into his scrotal sac. Sometimes one or both testicles don't descend, and the boy has what doctors call an *undescended testicle*. (At times, cold weather, a cold bath, excitement, or extreme physical activity will cause one or both of a boy's testicles to retract, that is, to draw up close to his body for a while. But this is a temporary conditon. It's not the same as an undescended testicle.)

No one knows what causes an undescended testicle, but luckily doctors do know how to cure it. Sometimes the doctor can use medicine to make the testicle descend; at other times it's necessary for the boy to have an operation.

This is really embarrassing, so you'd better keep your promise about not letting anyone see these questions 'cause someone might know my handwriting. This is what happened. I was masturbating and I didn't want to get it all over my pj's, so I put my finger over the top of my penis just as I was going to come so nothing would come out. And nothing did, but for the last couple of days I've had this pain in my penis and this milky stuff has come out. What should I do?

First of all, I always keep my promise, and no one in the class (or me, for that matter) had any idea who wrote this question. Second, this kind of problem is not at all unusual among boys. It's called *retrograde ejaculation*, and it happens when the semen is prevented from spurting out the opening in the glans of the penis during ejaculation. In older men, there are certain medical problems that cause retrograde ejaculation. But in boys, it usually happens when the boy is masturbating, and for some reason or another doesn't want to ejaculate. So he puts his hand or thumb or something over the opening in the penis as he's about to ejaculate, as the boy who asked this question did.

Retrograde means "going backward." In retrograde ejaculation, the semen can't come out the end of the penis, so it travels backward down the urethra. It may be forced up the tube that leads to the bladder, which can cause the urine to be cloudy for some time afterward. The semen may also be forced into the prostate gland. In either case, there may be pain and discharge from the penis.

In some instances, the symptoms will clear up all by themselves, but often a doctor's care is needed. Al-

retrograde (RET-row-grade)

though it may be embarrassing for a boy to tell the doctor that he's been masturbating and to explain how the retrograde ejaculation happened, it's important to see the doctor if you have pain, a milky discharge, or milky urine. If the semen is forced up into the prostate gland, the tissues of the gland could become irritated and susceptible to infection. The doctor can treat such infections with antibiotics and, if necessary, with pain-killers.

I'm not circumcised, and my penis is kind of swollen and red and stuck, so I can't pull it down. What's wrong?
Sometimes boys who haven't been circumcised develop these kinds of symptoms. They are caused by a foreskin that's too tight or foreskin that becomes stuck to the glans of the penis. This can be quite uncomfortable and can cause pain and swelling. Such problems are usually cured by circumcision. If you are dead set against circumcision, there are other ways of treating the problem. It's important, though, that you see a doctor and have the problem taken care of.

I have pain in my genitals, but I don't really want to see a doctor. I've never had sex, so it can't be VD. What could it be?
It's a bit difficult to say what could be causing this problem without knowing more. We've already explained about urethritis, retrograde ejaculation, and foreskin problems in uncircumcised boys, any of which could cause pain in the genitals. In addition, here are some other possibilities.

- Swollen glands: There are certain glands in the genital area called lymph glands. It's possible, even if you've never had sex, to get an infection in these glands, which

lymph (LIMF)

can cause pain and swelling. Treatment with antibiotics usually cures the problem.

- "Blue balls": "Blue balls" isn't really a disease or a medical problem, but it can cause pain or an achy feeling in the testicles or genital area. Blue balls happens when a boy has an erection for a long time without ejaculating or without having his penis get soft again (because he's still sexually stimulated). For example, a boy could have a long kissing session with his girlfriend that could cause him to have a prolonged erection that might result in blue balls. Even after his erection goes away, the achy feeling may persist. It happens because the blood is trapped in the penis for such a long time. Although it may be uncomfortable for a while, it's not a serious problem and doesn't require a doctor's treatment. The achy feeling goes away in, at most, a few hours.

- Hernia: A hernia occurs when part of the intestines bulge through a weak spot in the wall of the abdomen. If it happens in the lower part of the abdomen, it can cause pain in the genital area. If untreated, hernias can cause serious medical problems. They are usually treated by surgery in which the doctor repairs the weak spot.

- Twisted testicles: No one knows just why this happens; it is rare, but when it does occur it is a medical emergency. It usually follows some physical exertion and causes extreme pain, nausea, vomiting, and fever. It requires immediate surgery to correct.

I have these funny pimples (white) on my penis.
I've never had sex. Why does this happen?

You can't get VD, or sexually transmitted diseases, unless you have some sort of sexual contact with another person. But the skin of your penis, just like the skin on other parts of your body, is subject to all sorts of pimples, bumps, warts, irritations, birthmarks, scars, and so forth. The white, pimplelike bumps this boy describes are probably just blocked oil glands in the skin of his penis. Such pimples aren't anything to worry about. Of

hernia (HER-knee-eh)

course, if you have some problem that bothers you, it's always a good idea to have it checked out by your doctor.

I have this lump in my scrotum. It doesn't hurt, but it's there. What is it? Can guys get cancer of the scrotum?
Most lumps or bumps in the scrotum are the result of cysts, collections of fluid. Some of these cysts will go away all by themselves. Some require an operation. Although the vast majority of lumps in boys' scrotums are not serious, it's a good idea to get them checked out by a doctor.

It is possible for boys to get cancer of the testicles and scrotum, but it is very rare. When it does happen, the first symptom is often a lump in the scrotum. This doesn't mean that *all* lumps (or even most lumps) in the scrotal sac are cancerous lumps. But because a few are, it's important to have any lump checked out by a doctor. Although it can happen to older and younger men, testicle cancer is most often found in young men between the ages of twenty and thirty-five. The earlier it is found, the easier it is to cure. For this reason, doctors recommend that boys and men practice a regular testicular self-exam, which is explained in Illustration 32.

SEXUAL CRIMES

Since we're talking about sexuality and problems associated with sexuality, it's important that we also talk about sexual crimes. Parents are sometimes reluctant to bring up the topic of sexual crimes with their children because they don't want to scare them. They want to protect their children from even hearing about such

cysts (SISTS)

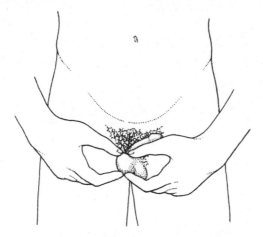

Illustration 32. Testicular self-exam. It's best to examine your scrotum right after a hot bath or shower. The scrotal skin is most relaxed at this time, and the testicles can be felt more easily. Examine each gently with the fingers of both hands. Put your index and middle fingers on the under side of the testicle and your thumb on the top. Roll your testicle gently between your thumb and fingers, feeling for a small lump about the size of a pea. Repeat this procedure for the other testicle.

You should learn what the epididymis feels like at the back of the testicle so that you won't confuse it with an abnormality. If you do find anything abnormal, most often it will be a firm area on the front or side of the testicle.

Testicular cancer constitutes fewer than 1 percent of all cancers, but it is one of the most common cancers in men aged twenty to thirty-five years. It's forty times more likely to occur among men in whom the testes never descend to the scrotum or descend after the age of six.

Most testicular cancers are first discovered by men themselves. Since testicular cancers found early and treated promptly have an excellent chance for cure, learning how to examine your testes properly can help save your life. It really doesn't take much effort to search for those small lumps, and you only have to do it once a month. Use the simple testicular self-examination (TSE) procedure shown here.

terrible things. This is understandable, but the fact of the matter is, sexual crimes do happen. We feel that the best way to protect children from sexual crimes is to make sure they know about these things and are prepared to handle the situation if they become victims of a sexual crime.

The three types of sexual crimes we will be talking about here are rape, incest, and child molesting. *Rape* means forcing someone to have sex against his or her will. It can happen to anyone—to young kids, to adults, to people of any age. Most rape victims are females, and most rapists are males. Theoretically, it's possible for a woman to hold a gun to a man's head and force him to have intercourse with her, or for a woman to force a person (male or female) to have oral-genital sex with her, or something like this. And probably somewhere in the world at some time such things have happened. It is also possible for a man to be raped by another man. By and large, though, rape cases involve a male raping a female.

Incest involves one member of a family being sexual with another family member. It may include anything from touching, feeling, or kissing the sex organs to actual sexual intercourse. Of course, it isn't incest when a husband and wife do these things with each other. But when it happens between other family members, it's called incest.

Most victims of incest are girls who are victimized by their fathers, stepfathers, brothers, uncles, cousins, or some other male relative, although it is also possible for a girl to be victimized by a female relative. Boys can also be victims of incest, but this is less common. When incest happens to a boy, it may be either a female or a male relative who victimizes him. Incest can happen to very young children, even to babies, as well as to older kids and teenagers.

Brothers and sisters often engage in some form of sex play as they're growing up, which may involve "playing doctor" or "pretending to be mommy and daddy" and trying out sex. This kind of sex play between brothers and sisters is very common and isn't always considered incest. It isn't necessarily a harmful thing. But being forced or pressured to have sexual contact with an older brother or sister *is* incest, and it can be very harmful.

Incest isn't always a forced thing, like rape. Because of the older person's position in the family, he (or she) may be able to pressure the child into doing sexual things without actually having to use force. Most incest victims are so bewildered by what's going on that they simply don't know how to stop it or prevent it from happening again.

Child molesting, like incest, may involve anything from touching, feeling, or kissing the sex organs to actual sexual intercourse. (The word *molest* means to bother or to harm.) But child molesting is different from incest because the person doing the molesting isn't a family member. It may be a complete stranger, a friend of the child's parents, or some other older person. Boys as well as girls may be victims of a child molester.

If you are a victim of a sexual crime, the most important thing to do is *tell someone.* This can be a difficult thing to do, particularly if you are a victim of incest or child molesting. The logical people to tell are your parents. However, it's not always easy for parents to believe their children at first. If you feel your parents won't believe you, for whatever reason, you might tell another relative—an aunt or uncle, a grandparent, an older sister or brother—who you feel *will* believe you. Or you could tell another adult—a teacher or counselor at school, a friend's mom or dad, your minister or priest, or any other adult you trust. You can also call a rape hotline, which will help you no matter what sexual crime you have been a victim of. Most big cities, and other smaller ones, have these kinds of hotlines, and they are listed under the heading "rape" in the phone book. Or you can call the nearest hospital and ask to talk to the doctor in charge of the emergency room or a doctor from the pediatrics (children's medicine) department. You can also call or go to the police station and tell a police officer.

Telling someone is also hard because incest and child molesting are crimes, and it's possible that your telling could get the person who's been victimizing you into legal trouble. But you should know that most people who commit incest aren't sent to jail. (*Victims* of these crimes are not criminals, and victims are *never* punished legally.) If at all possible, the judge, the social worker, or whoever is in charge arranges for the person who's been committing the crime to get some sort of psychiatric help or treatment.

Some incest victims hesitate to tell because they're afraid that the family will break up, that their parents will get divorced, or that things will just get worse than they are already. But if incest is going on, things are already about as bad as they could be. People who commit incest are sick mentally, but they can be cured. The victim and other family members also need help in dealing with the situation. But no one can help unless the victim has enough courage to take the first step and let someone know what's happening.

pediatrics (pee-dee-AT-trix)

Most victims of incest and child molesting feel a mixture of embarrassment, guilt, and shame. This can also make it hard to come forward and tell someone. But you have a right to protect yourself from being touched in ways that don't feel right to you. So even though you may feel embarrassed, it's important to tell someone. It's really the best thing for everyone.

OTHER QUESTIONS

We hope we've answered most of your questions, but there are probably some things you've wondered about that we haven't covered. If so, perhaps your dad or mom, the school nurse, one of your teachers, or another adult can help you find answers. Or, as we explained at the end of Chapter 1, you can always write to us. Our address is listed on page 42.

CHAPTER 8

A Few Final Words

As you know, there are a number of physical changes that take place in our bodies during puberty. For most of us, these physical changes are accompanied by certain emotional changes. For instance, we may feel very "up," proud, and excited about the fact that we're growing up and becoming adults. But along with these positive feelings, most of us also experience less-than-totally-wonderful feelings from time to time as we're going through puberty. It's not uncommon for young people to have the "blues," times when we feel depressed or down in the dumps, sometimes for no apparent reason. Part of the reason we have these feelings may be the new hormones our bodies are making. Hormones are powerful substances, and they can affect our emotions. It takes our bodies and emotions some time to adjust to these hormones, and some doctors feel that the emotional ups and downs many young people experience are due, at least in part, to hormonal changes. But it's undoubtedly more than that. It's not just our bodies that are changing, it's our whole lives. At times, all this changing can seem a bit over-whelming, and we may feel uncertain, scared, anxious, or depressed.

One girl wrote to my daughter and me after she'd read the girl's book on puberty, expressing feelings that a lot of kids share. She said:

> I'm going through puberty now and I'm very scared about it. Everyone says it's normal to feel this way, but every time I'm feeling good and everything, I suddenly get this de-pressed feeling and I don't want to grow up anymore. I just never want to get older and face things like possible rapes, diseases, deaths, etc.
>
> Also, I'm going into my first year of junior high school and I'm really scared. I'm not sure I'm ready to face all the changes.

It is quite normal to have these kinds of feelings. Knowing that other kids your age have the same feel-ings won't magically make you feel better, but it can help you to know that at least you're not alone.

Sometimes, young people are upset because they feel pressured to grow up all at once. As one boy put it:

> Everyone I know is trying to grow up as fast as possible. What's the rush? I'm just not in a great big rush. I want to take my time. I'm tired of everyone trying to act all big and grown-up all the time.

And sometimes, the idea of being more grown-up and independent can be kind of scary. As one boy said:

> Okay, so now all of a sudden I'm supposed to be all grown-up and have all these adult responsibilities. But I'm not ready to have these responsibilities and make all these

decisions. In a few years, I'm going to go to college or maybe
get a job and live on my own, and I don't know even what I
want to do or if I can really do everything on my own. Sometimes I just want to stay a little kid.

However, there may be times when we feel that people around us, especially our parents, are keeping us
from growing up as fast as we'd like to. One teenage
girl expressed this point of view:

Sometimes I really hate my parents. They treat me like a
little kid. They want to tell me what to wear or how I should
wear my hair and where I can go and who I can go with and
when I have to be home and blah, blah, blah. They're always
bugging me. It's like they want me to stay "their little girl"
forever and they won't let me grow up.

Going through puberty and becoming a teenager
doesn't necessarily mean that you and your parents will
have problems getting along with each other, but most
teens do run into at least some conflicts with their parents. Indeed, at times it can seem like out-and-out war.
These conflicts between teens and parents have to do
with the change that takes place in the relationship
between the parent and child during these years. When
we're little babies, we can't even feed ourselves, change
our clothes, or go to the bathroom by ourselves. Our
parents have to feed us, dress us, and change our
diapers; we are *dependent* on them for everything. It's
our parents' job to teach us how to take care of ourselves so that, eventually, we'll be able to go out and
live on our own. And they have to take care of us and
protect us until we're old enough to do that for ourselves. Children need their parents, but they also want
to grow up, to be more independent, to take care of
themselves, and to make decisions on their own. At the

beginning of your teen years, you are still very dependent, but in a few years you'll be off to college or out earning your own living. So during your teen years, you and your parents are ending a relationship in which you're very dependent, and trying to establish a new relationship in which you are totally independent.

It's not easy to let go of old, familiar ways of relating and to establish new ones. Parents are used to being in charge, to making decisions. They may continue to tell you how to dress, how to wear your hair, what to do and when to do it, even after you feel that you're old enough to make these decisions on your own. This change in the relationship from dependent to independent doesn't usually come off without a hitch, and much of the stress, anger, and other negative feelings that you may experience during your teen years have to do with a working out of the change in the relationship with your parents.

Our relationships with our friends also change during these years, and here again, this changing can cause uncertain, confused, depressed, or otherwise difficult emotional feelings. Chances are you'll begin junior high and be going to a new school, making new friends, perhaps seeing less of old friends. Breaking old ties and making new ones isn't always an easy thing to do. During these years, being part of a certain gang or group usually becomes a very important part of your life. It can make things easier and more fun. But groups can present problems, too. You may find that you aren't accepted into a certain "in" group even though you'd like very much to be part of it. Feelings of being "out of it" or being excluded from the group can make things seem very lonely.

Even if you are accepted by the group, you may find that there are still some problems. Being part of a group can have a lot of rewards—it helps us feel more accepted, more a part of things, less lonely and uncertain. But sometimes being part of the group "costs" us. We may have to act in certain ways or do certain things we don't feel good about doing in order to stay part of the group. Here's what some kids had to say about this:

> I really want to be "in" with this group of kids at school, but they do some things I don't like. Like they're always laughing at kids who aren't in the group, making jokes or comments and stuff when one of those kids gets up in front of class or something. I really want to be accepted, and it's like I have to do what they do to be accepted. But if I do, I don't feel good about myself.
>
> Margie, age 14

> I hate school 'cause I either have to act a certain way or be some outcast. Like in class, if you have an idea about something that is different from everyone else's, you can't say it or you'll be out of it and everyone will put you down. You have to do and say the same thing as everyone else or you're not okay.
>
> Tim, age 13

> Friends can talk me into doing things I don't really want to do. I'm in with the really "in" crowd, but the kids I run around with drink and smoke dope 'cause that's cool. My parents would kill me if they knew what I do, and really I'm not so into these things, but I do them to be part of the group.
>
> Sharon, age 15

This business of being part of the group isn't a problem for all teenagers, but it is for many. Another change that many kids find difficult and that can cause emotional problems is the change in the relationships between boys and girls that usually takes place during these years. Sometimes, it seems that all the rules have suddenly changed. The kids in my ten- to twelve year old class usually have a lot to say about this. Here's what one boy said:

> I'm going to Jennifer's halloween party on Saturday, and my sister keeps teasing me, "Oh, you like Jennifer, you're in love with Jennifer." Well, I do like Jennifer, but not like that. It's now, all of a sudden, you can't just be friends with a girl. It's got to be boyfriend and girlfriend, like you're all romantic with each other.
>
> Tom, age 12

Another boy and girl, I'll call them Donny and Hillary, who've been friends since they were little kids, had this to say:

> I went over to Hillary's house to spend the night, and we were swimming in the pool. These girls who live next door came over and they were saying things like, "Oh, you're playing with a girl. Oh, you're staying overnight at a girl's house. Oh, that's weird. You must be gay."
>
> Donny, age 11

> Yeah, then they realized they'd seen Donny on TV in that movie he was in. Then they started acting all different— "Ohh, you're sooo cute," and trying to act all sexy. Then they made it like he was my boyfriend, and it was all different than when he was just going to stay overnight at my house.
>
> Hillary, age 11

We may find that our feelings about the opposite sex are changing. We may develop a crush on someone. Crushes can be fun, but they can also be very painful, especially if the other person doesn't feel the same way we do.

Once you begin dating, you may find yourself having

to make decisions about how you are going to handle sexuality. As we discussed in Chapter 7, making these kinds of decisions is not an easy thing to do.

Growing up is indeed a mixed bag of experiences. On the one hand, there are a lot of exciting things to look forward to; on the other hand, there are a lot of changes —physical changes, life changes, changes in our relationships with our parents, our friends, and with the opposite sex. Probably at some time there must have been someone, somewhere, who went through puberty and the teenage years without a single problem, but we wouldn't bet a whole lot of money on it. If you're like most kids, you'll run into some problems as you go through the physical and emotional changes of puberty. We hope that this book will help you in dealing with these problems. But this book is only a beginning. In the next section, we've included a list of some other books we think you'll find helpful.

FOR FURTHER READING

BOOKS FOR YOUNG CHILDREN

Ideally sex education should begin at a very early age. One way to introduce the topic is through one of the excellent picture books for young children. The following are among our favorites and are appropriate for four- to eight-year-olds.

DRAGONWAGON, CRESCENT. *Windrose* (New York: Harper & Row, 1976).

A lovely, lyrical picture book in which a mother describes to her child how the child was conceived and how it felt to carry the child and give birth. A nurturing, loving story that, although it doesn't explain the sex act explicitly, puts forth the notion that sex is a wonderful, beautiful feeling.

GORDON, SOL and JUDITH. *Did the Sun Shine Before You Were Born?* (New York: Okapaku Publishing, Inc., 1974).

This book is multiethnic and nonsexist, and it presents a variety of different families. It deals with the topics of sexuality, conception, pregnancy, and birth in clear, simple terms.

SHEFFIELD, MARGARET. *Where Do Babies Come From?* (New York: Knopf, 1978).

This book explains puberty, sex, conception, pregnancy, and birth in terms that even a very young child can understand. It is sensitively done and beautifully illustrated. Possibly the best single introductory sex-education book for young readers.

WAXMAN, STEPHANIE. *What is a Girl? What is a Boy?* (Los Angeles: Peace Press, 1976).

This frank and forthright book, illustrated with nude photos of infants, children, and adults, deals with the physical differences between sexes. Nonsexist and sensitive, it deals with typical children's questions, such as, "Will I grow one?", "Will mine fall off?", "Will I always be a girl/boy?" Although marred by the curious fact that the author refers to the vulva as the vagina, this is, nonetheless, an excellent book.

BOOKS FOR TEENS

Austin, Al and Hefner, Keith, eds. *Growing Up Gay* (Ann Arbor: Youth Liberation Press, 1978).

This collection of essays, written by gay young people, deals with the issues homosexuals face as they are growing up. To order, send $1.75 to Youth Liberation Press, 2007 Washington Avenue, Ann Arbor, Michigan 48104.

BELL, RUTH. *Changing Bodies, Changing Lives: A Book for Teens on Sex and Relationships* (New York: Random House, 1981).

Absolutely the best book for teens on the topic, representing many points of view through quotes from teenagers themselves. The first section deals with the physical changes of puberty, including how it feels to have a wet dream, a first period, and so on. The next section deals with interpersonal issues between parents and teens, and teens and peers—as well as loneliness, love, marriage, divorce, and sex-role expectations. The middle two sections of the book are devoted to sexuality and cover masturbation, sexual fantasies, kissing, petting, oral-genital sex, intercourse, and sexual problems, without taking a specific stand on moral issues. There is also an excellent section on rape and incest and good information on drugs and alcohol, sexually transmitted diseases, and birth control. The section on teenage pregnancy is especially good, and the one on mental health, depression, and suicide is outstanding. The book is geared toward the fourteen- to nineteen-year-old age group, but it could be valuable for younger and older people as well.

CALDERONE, MARY S., M.D. and JOHNSON, ERIC W. *The Family Book about Sexuality*, rev. ed. (New York: Bantam Books, 1983).

This book is designed for the whole family. It talks about how sexuality begins when we are only tiny babies, and how it develops through puberty and adulthood. It also covers sexuality and old people. It has lots of good information about love and marriage, birth control, and sexual problems. It should be part of every family's book collection.

COMFORT, ALEX and JANE. *The Facts of Love: Living, Loving, and Growing* (New York: Crown, 1979).

This book covers many of the same topics dealt with in *Changing Bodies, Changing Lives*, and it is especially good for younger adolescents (ages ten to thirteen). The illustrations are lovely. More conservative parents may be more comfortable with this book than with the much franker presentation in *Changing Bodies*; however, in my experience, teens themselves much prefer Bell's book. Parents who worry that presenting information about sexuality to their children might lead to promiscuous behavior owe it to themselves to read the introduction to *The Facts of Love*.

THE DIAGRAM GROUP. *Man's Body: An Owner's Manual* (New York: Bantam Books, 1977).

This is an excellent book that has a chapter on the male sex organs and one on sexuality. It also covers other parts of the body, illness, body care, fitness, food, drugs, aging, and just about anything an owner of a male body would want to know.

THE DIAGRAM GROUP. *Sex: A User's Manual* (New York: Berkley, 1982).

This is an extremely straightforward, up-to-date guide that covers virtually every aspect of sexual experience, sexual development, and social attitudes about sex, including methods of intercourse, the phases of sexual excitement, foreplay, orgasm, unconventional sex practices, sexual problems, sex crimes, and prostitution. It also discusses attraction and courtship, birth control, and sexually transmitted diseases. The book is aimed at an adult audience, but the information is presented in a well-illustrated format and is written in clear, simple prose that teens can readily understand. Again, more conservative parents may feel uncomfortable with this book because it deals so openly with the varieties of sexual behavior.

GARDNER-LOULAN, JOANN; LOPEZ, BONNIE; and QUACKENBUSH, MARIA. *Period* (San Francisco: Volcano Press, 1981).

The excellent picture book deals with menstruation and is especially useful for introducing preteens to the topic. The illustrations, which feature all ethnic groups and even handicapped kids (which most books don't do), are marvelous and depict all types of girls, not just conventionally pretty, idealized body types. Although it is written for young girls, it is also worthwhile for young boys.

MADARAS, LYNDA and AREA. *What's Happening to My Body?: A Growing Up Guide for Mothers and Daughters.* (New York: Newmarket Press, 1983).

This is the book my daughter and I wrote for girls about puberty. Needless to say, we think it's a pretty good one. Although it was written for girls, many boys and parents have read it and told us they learned a lot from it.

MCCOY, KATHY and WIBBELSMAN, CHARLES, M.D. *The Teenage Body Book* (New York: Simon and Schuster, 1981).

This is a good source book for older teens, and it covers some topics, such as plastic surgery, medical problems teens may have, and sports injuries, that aren't dealt with in many other books.

PLANNED PARENTHOOD. *Kids Need to Know.*

Kids Need to Know is an information kit for parents and teens. It contains the booklet "Let's Talk About . . . S-E-X," by Sam Gitchel and Lorri Foster, and a number of pamphlets such as "Teen Sex?: It's OK to Say No Way" and "Basics of Birth Control." The kit is available for $10.00 (which includes postage and handling) from the Information and Education Department, Planned Parenthood, 1920 Marengo Street, Los Angeles, California 90033.

POMERY, WARDELL. *Boys and Sex* and *Girls and Sex* (New York: Dell, 1982).

These two books, first written in 1968, have recently been rereleased. The first chapter in each book covers anatomy. The later chapters deal with masturbation, homosexuality, dating, petting, intercourse, and the consequences of intercourse. Some people may disagree with some of the attitudes toward homosexuality, and parts of the book seem a bit dated. On the whole, though, these are excellent books.

INDEX

Lynda Madaras lectures frequently on healthcare subjects and teaches coed classes in puberty and sex and health education to teens and preteens in Santa Monica, California. Her book *What's Happening to My Body?: A Growing Up Guide for Mothers and Daughters*, which she wrote with her daughter, Area, was named a 1983 Best Book for Young Adults by the American Library Association. She is the author of *Child's Play* and coauthor of *Womancare, Great Expectations, The Alphabet Connection,* and *Woman/Doctor: The Education of Jane Patterson, M.D.*

Dane Saavedra, who collaborated on this book with Lynda Madaras, is a fifteen-year-old high school student and the son of one of Madaras's long-time friends.

Available in both gift hardcover and trade paperback

THE "WHAT'S HAPPENING TO MY BODY?" BOOK
FOR BOYS
A Growing Up Guide for Parents and Sons
Lynda Madaras with Dane Saavedra

Also available, for girls:
WHAT'S HAPPENING TO MY BODY?
A Growing Up Guide for Mothers and Daughters
Lynda Madaras with Area Madaras

This carefully researched book provides detailed explanations of what takes place in a girl's body as she grows up, and includes chapters on: changing size and shape • changes in the reproductive organs • the menstrual cycle • puberty in boys • and much more. Includes over 40 drawings, bibliography, index.

"Supportive, down-to-earth"—*Publishers Weekly*

"The beauty of this book is the absolutely natural way Madaras encourages the young woman to explore, understand and accept her own special body at the same time she is learning the basic facts of female development."—SIECUS Report

A "Best Book for Young Adults, 1983"—American Library Association

**Ask for these titles at your local bookstore or
Order Today**

Use this coupon or write to: NEWMARKET PRESS, 3 East 48th Street, New York, New York, 10017.

Please send me:
_____ copies of WHAT'S HAPPENING TO MY BODY? @ $14.95 (gift hardcover)
_____ copies of WHAT'S HAPPENING TO MY BODY? @ $8.95 (trade paperback)
_____ copies of THE "WHAT'S HAPPENING TO MY BODY?" BOOK FOR BOYS @ $14.95 (gift hardcover)
_____ copies of THE "WHAT'S HAPPENING TO MY BODY?" BOOK FOR BOYS @ $8.95 (trade paperback)

Add $1.50 per order for postage and handling. Allow 4–6 weeks for delivery. (NY residents, please add applicable state and local sales tax.)

I enclose check or money order payable to NEWMARKET PRESS in the amount of $_____.

NAME _____
ADDRESS _____
CITY/STATE/ZIP _____

For quotes on quantity purchases, or for a copy of our catalog, please write or phone Newmarket Press, 3 East 48th Street, New York, N.Y. 10017. 1-212-832-3575.